ONCOGENESIS, INFLAMMATORY AND PARASITIC TROPICAL DISEASES OF THE LUNG

Edited by **Jean-Marie Kayembe**

Oncogenesis, Inflammatory and Parasitic Tropical Diseases of the Lung
http://dx.doi.org/10.5772/56085
Edited by Jean-Marie Kayembe

Contributors

Luis Antón Aparicio, Sergio Vazquez Estevez, Jean-Marie Kayembe, Benjamin Longo-Mbenza, Matthew Thomas Hardison, Kazushi Inoue, Sinan Zhu, Gil, Marta Adonis, Ahmet Baydur, Menno Van Der Eerden, S Uzun

Published by InTech
Janeza Trdine 9, 51000 Rijeka, Croatia

Publishing Process Manager Viktorija Zgela
Technical Editor InTech DTP team
Cover InTech Design team

Additional hard copies can be obtained from orders@intechopen.com

Oncogenesis, Inflammatory and Parasitic Tropical Diseases of the Lung, Edited by Jean-Marie Kayembe
p. cm.
ISBN 978-953-51-0982-2

For EU product safety concerns:
IN TECH d.o.o., Prolaz Marije Krucifikse Kozulić 3, 51000 Rijeka, Croatia,
info@intechopen.com or visit our website at intechopen.com.

Meet the editor

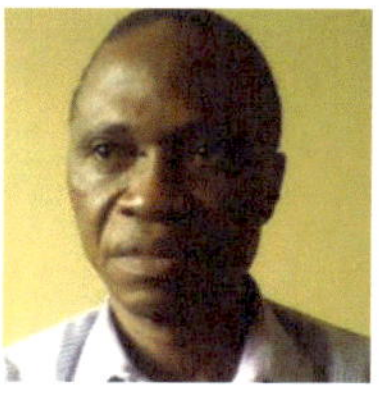

Jean-Marie KAYEMBE Ntumba, MD, PhD
Professor of Pneumology, Faculty of Medicine, University of Kinshasa/ D R Congo
Editor of Annales Africaines de Médecine
Coordinator of SACIDS (Southern African Centre for infectious Disease Surveillance)
Member of European Respiratory Society; Société de Pneumologie de Langue Française (SPLF); SAPLF (Société Africaine de Pneumologie de Langue Française); Pan African Thoracic Society (PATS)
Honorary Deputy Dean/ Faculty of Medicine / Unikin
Chief of The Departement of Lung Diseases/ University Hospital of Kinshasa

Contents

Preface

In this book dealing with the lung health, the authors focus on various fields, spreading from pulmonary oncogenesis, to inflammatory and parasitic lung diseases.

The first section deals with the fundamental research on lung cancer that is mandatory for the development of novel and early biomarkers for diagnosis of the lung cancer. This development could be enhanced using experimental models despite the species barrier. Mouse models can help us understand the sequence of events involved in human lung neoplasia and their underlying molecular mechanisms.

The results of the research could be used to identify novel targets for the development of new biological therapies.

In the second section of this book, the role of inflammation in various respiratory diseases is outlined. The authors recall cellular mechanisms including neutrophils to improve the understanding of the phenomenon and help develop targeted therapies.

The third section on parasitic tropical lung disease highlights the growing importance of neglected tropical diseases due to increased traffic across the continents and migration of the population. Physicians need to be aware of the symptoms and imaging findings of these diseases mainly in travelers and immigrants from tropical endemic areas.

Jean-Marie Kayembe

Section 1

Oncogenesis and the Lung

Chapter 1

Angiogenesis and Lung Cancer

S. Vázquez, U. Anido, M. Lázaro, L. Santomé,
J. Afonso, O. Fernández, A. Martínez de Alegría and
L. A. Aparicio

Additional information is available at the end of the chapter

http://dx.doi.org/10.5772/54309

1. Introduction

Angiogenesis is the formation of new blood vessels from the existing vasculature, and neovascularization is a prerequisite for the growth of solid tumors beyond 1-2 mm in diameter [1]. Because of this, during tumorigenesis, tumor growth reaches a growth-limiting step where oxygen and nutrient levels are insufficient to continue proliferation.

Tumors acquire blood vessels by co-option of neighboring vessels from sprouting or intussuscepted microvascular growth and by vasculogenesis from endothelial precursor cells [2]. In most solid tumors the newly formed vessels are plagued by structural and functional abnormalities due to the sustained and excessive exposure to angiogenic factors produced by the tumor [3]. As a result of this, the new tumor-associated vasculature is abnormal and inefficient, but it is essential for tumor growth and metastasis. Despite being abnormal, these new vessels allow tumor growth at early stages of carcinogenesis and progression from in situ lesions to locally invasive, and eventually to metastatic tumors.

As a result, tumors tend to become hypoxic. The normal cellular response to hypoxia is to produce growth factors such as vascular endothelial growth factor (VEGF), transforming growth factor alpha (TGF-α), and platelet derived growth factor (PDGF), by neoplastic, stromal cells or inflammatory cells [4], and may trigger an angiogenic switch to allow the tumor to induce the formation of microvessels from the surrounding host vasculature [5], that stimulate neoangiogenesis [6].

VEGF is the most potent and specific growth factor for endothelial cells, and is associated with tumor vessel density, cancer metastasis, and prognosis [7-10]: high levels of circulating VEGF have been reported in patients with non-small cell lung cancer (NSCLC)

[7,10-18]. VEGF is continuously expressed throughout the development of many tumor types, and is the only angiogenic factor known to be present throughout the entire tumor life cycle [19]. The clinical significance of circulating levels of VEGF in patients with NSCLC is controversial.

Since tumor growth and metastasis are angiogenesis-dependent, relying upon the generation of new blood vessels to sustain proliferation, survival and spread of the malignant cells, therapeutic strategies aimed at inhibiting angiogenesis area theoretically attractive. Targeting and damaging blood vessels can potentially kill thousands of tumor cells. The antiangiogenesis and vascular targeting strategies, therefore, may no result in whole tumor cell kill, but may maintain stable disease: this has given rise to the concept *cytostatic paradigm* [20].

The investigation and development of different anti-angiogenesis and vascular targeting strategies are of interest with respect to lung cancer.

2. Hypoxia and lung cancer, HIF-1α, carbonic anhydrase IX and glucose transporter glut

Hypoxia is one of the most important challenges for tumor growth and survival. The angiogenesis is a fundamental to avoid tumor necrosis (TN); every cell in a tissue is forced to be within 100μm capillary blood vessel [5].

Hypoxia inducible factor-1 (HIF-1) is a regulator of VEGF under hypoxia conditions [21].

HIF-1 is a heterodimer consisting of 2 subunits, HIF-1α and HIF-1β (otherwise known as the aryl hydrocarbon receptor nuclear translocator), which is stabilized by hypoxia. The expression of these subunits is different; HIF-1β is constitutively expressed, unlike HIF-1α, which is rapidly degraded under normoxic conditions [22]. In the presence of oxygen, HIF-1α is hydroxylated on conserved prolyl residues within the oxygen-dependent degradation domain by prolylhydroxylases and binds to von Hippel-Lindau protein (pVHL), which in turn targets it for degradation through the ubiquitin-proteasome pathway [23-26]. Hypoxia inhibits hydroxylation of prolyl residues 402 and 564 in the oxygen-dependent degradation domain that avoid binding of the pVHL. Similar hypoxia-dependent inhibition of hydroxylation of asparagines residues within the C-terminal activation domain increases HIF-1α transcriptional activity. Oxygen-dependent degradation of HIF-1α is inhibited by *src* and *ras* oncogenes [22-25].

The HIF-1 complex recognizes hypoxia response elements on the promoter of several genes, including VEGF, PDGF, and TGF-α [26].

Growth factors, cytokines and oncogenes, which stimulate p42/p44 mitogen-associated protein kinase (MAPK) and/or phosphoinositidyl-3 kinase (PI-3K) pathways, may enhance HIF-1 activity. HIF-1 binds to a conserved sequence (5-CGTG-3) known as the hypoxic response element in the promoter region of its target genes. These target genes are involved in processes that promote cellular survival, angiogenesis, blood vessel vasodilatation, erythropoiesis, anaerobic metabolism, buffering of the intracellular compartment and induction of growth factors. HIF-1 activity *in vivo* promotes tumor growth in the most of the studies and resistance to several chemotherapy agents, as platinum compounds [22]. Carbonic anhydrase (CA) IX and glucose transporter-1 are other transcriptional targets of HIF-1 and, along with HIF-1, have been identified as novel markers of hypoxia in different tumor types [27-31]. Up-regulation of CA IX in vivo in a perinecrotic pattern suggests this may be an important pathway in hypoxia, possibly regulating pH to allow survival of cells under hypoxic conditions [28].

Other study showed that HIF-1 is commonly expressed in NSCLC and is involved in the pathogenesis of NSCLC. HIF-1 expression seems associated with a poor prognosis and this was found to be as an independent factor. A similar observation has been made for the prognostic impact of the extent of TN, another marker for hypoxia in NSCLC, where although extensive TN predicts outcome in earlier stages of the disease, no such effect is seen in locally advanced disease. Thus, a number of other studies have included patients with locally advanced disease in different cancer types and reported an association between HIF-1 expression and prognosis [22]. Although some other studies have reported different results [32].

The associations between HIF-1, CA IX, TN and squamous NSCLC are coherent with the known pathways that regulate and are regulated by HIF-1. CA IX is regulated by HIF-1. TN and CA IX have been associated with a poor prognosis in NSCLC [22,31].

By other hand, glucose transporter GLUT-1 is a potential intrinsic marker of hypoxia in cancer [29]. VEGF and GLUT-1 are similarly regulated in response to hypoxia [33]. They may functionally help each other to endure hypoxia. Therefore, an upregulated expression of GLUT-1 allows the cell to better use an inadequate source of glucose, while an upregulated expression of VEGF will improve the reserve of glucose and oxygen through the recruitment of additional blood vessels [33].

3. Pathophysiology and clinical implications of VEGF

The role of angiogenesis in cancer biology was defended by Folkman in 1971, who first postulated that solid tumors remained latent at a specific size due to the absence of neovascularization, that was conditioned by the diffusion of oxygen and nutrients [34].

Subsequent studies have shown that angiogenesis is involved in tumor development from the initial stages to the most advanced stages of the disease [35]. Angiogenesis plays therefore, an important role in tumor growth and metastasis development.

Since then, one of the most important questions has been the identification of proangiogenic factors and the mechanisms in order to block its action. One of the most studied has been the VEGF.

VEGF is a potent mediator of angiogenesis. It is a growth factor that stimulates the proliferation and migration, promotes survival, inhibits apoptosis and regulates the permeability of vascular endothelial cells. It belongs to the growth factors family, which includes four homologues VEGF-A (commonly referred to as VEGF)-B, -C, -D, -E and placental growth factor (PIGF). The biological activity of VEGF is mediated by binding to receptors with tyrosine kinase activity VEGFR-1 (also known as fms-like tyrosine kinase 1, ftl-1), VEGFR-2 (also known as kinase-insert domain receptor, KDR) and VEGFR-3 (ftl4).

When VEGF binds to its receptors it causes receptor dimerization, autophosphorylation, and downstream signaling of different pathways, as v-src sarcoma viral oncogene homolog (Src), phosphoinositol (PI)-3 kinase (PI3K) and phospholipase-C γ (PLCγ) which activate proliferation and angiogenesis.

In animal tumor models, VEGF is produced both by tumor cells and also by stromal tissues [4].

VEGF and its receptor are expressed in tumor cells in both small cell lung cancer (SCLC) and non-small cell lung cancer (NSCLC) [36,37]. It is involved in tumor growth by neoangiogenesis, lymphangiogenesis and lymph nodal dissemination [38]. High levels of VEGF have been correlated with poor prognosis [39]. But there are several questions about the role of VEGF levels and its various isoforms plays as a potential biomarker, which may be useful in the use and selection of therapies against it. VEGF levels are elevated in lung cancer patients when compared to controls [40]. There is also a correlation between VEGF levels and the clinical stage in NSCLC patients [7,10,13,15] and an inverse correlation between the VEGF serum levels and survival [41]. Low levels of VEGF have shown to be correlated with a good response to chemotherapy [12]. Moreover, a study showed that low levels of VEGF were correlated with a good response to anti-EGFR. Furthermore, levels of VEGF in responders were not significantly different from volunteers, but were different from non-responders [42]. However, it remains unclear whether the clinical effects of anti-EGFR in patients with NSCLC are correlated with reductions in the levels of angiogenic growth factors. Furthermore, it is unclear whether these factors are correlated with response to anti-EGFR treatment, blocking EGFR autophosphorylation [43] and the subsequent signal transduction pathways implicated in proliferation, metastasis and inhibition of apoptosis, as well as angiogenesis [44,45]. The inhibition of EGFR has been shown to reduce production of angiogenic growth factors in various types of cancer cells [45,46].

Antiangiogenic drugs have demonstrated efficacy in the treatment of NSCLC in the last years. The more tested antiangiogenic drug in lung cancer is bevacizumab, a monoclonal antibody directed against VEGF, which is the first antiangiogenic approved for treatment of metastatic NSCLC in combination with chemotherapy. Two phase III studies have assessed the efficacy of chemotherapy combinations associated with bevacizumab. The AVAiL study [47] analyzed the combination of cisplatin and gemcitabine with or without bevacizumab in first line treatment for NSCLC. The primary endpoint was reached, showing a benefit in progression-free survival in the bevacizumab arm. The second study [48] compared the addition of bevacizumab with carboplatin and paclitaxel regimen, aiming differences in overall survival, progression-free survival and response rate.

These detailed studies further in subsequent chapters, show that bevacizumab is an effective and safe drug in the treatment of advanced NSCLC.

4. Pathophysiology and clinical implications of EGF/PDGF/VEG

It is known that other several growth factors regulate developmental processes, among which are the Epidermal Growth Factor (EGF), Fibroblast Growth Factor (FGF), growth factor Insulin-like type I (IGF-I) and Platelet Derived Growth Factor platelet (PDGF).

4.1. EGF

Members of the EGF family of peptide growth factors serve as agonists for ErbB family receptors. They include EGF, TGFα, amphiregulin (AR), betacellulin (BTC), heparin-binding EGF-like growth factor (HB-EGF), epiregulin (EPR), epigen (EPG), and the neuregulins (NRGs).

EGF is a polypeptide of 53 amino acids (6 Kda) that appears as a product of proteolytic processing of a large protein integral membrane (1207aa). This precursor protein is consisting of 8 domains called EGF-like, of which only one is active. The gene corresponding to this growth factor is located on chromosome 4q25 and stimulates epithelial cell proliferation, oncogenesis and is involved in wound healing. Its three-dimensional structure is characterized by the presence of common domain to other family ligands. This protein shows a strong sequential and functional homology with TGFα, which is a competitor for EGF receptor sites.

Collectively, these agonists regulate the activity of the four ErbB (Erythroblastic Leukemia Viral Oncogene Homolog) family receptors, each of which appears to make a unique set of contributions to a complicated signaling network.

EGF binds to a specific receptor on the surface of responsive cells known as EGFR (Epidermal growth factor receptor). EGFR is a member of the ErbB family receptors, a subfamily of four closely related to tyrosine kinase receptors: EGFR (ErbB1), Her2/c-neu (ErbB2), Her3 (ErbB3) and Her4 (ErbB4) (Fig.1). The EGF family ligands exhibits a complex pattern of interactions with the four ErbB family receptors; for example, EGFR can bind eight different EGF family members and Neuregulin 2beta (NRG2β) binds EGFR, ErbB3 and ErbB4. Given that ErbB2 lacks an EGF family ligand, ErbB3 lacks kinase activity, and the four ErbB receptor display distinct coupling patterns to different signaling effectors in the affinity of a given EGF family member as a key determinant of specificity for the ligand [49].

In response to toxic environmental stimuli, such as ultraviolet irradiation, or to receptor occupation by EGF, the EGFR forms Homo- or Heterodimers with other family members. Binding of EGF to the extracellular domain of EGFR leads to receptor dimerization, activation of the intrinsic PTK (Protein Tyrosine Kinase), tyrosine autophosphorylation, and recruitment of various signaling proteins to these autophosphorylation sites located primarily in the C-terminal tail of the receptor. Tyrosine phosphorylation of the EGFR leads to the recruitment of diverse signaling proteins, including the Adaptor proteins GRB2 (Growth Factor Receptor-Bound Protein-2) and Nck (Nck Adaptor Protein), PLC-&γ; (Phospholipase-C-γ), SHC (Src Homology-2 Domain Containing Transforming Protein), STATs (Signal Transducer and Activator of Transcription), and several other proteins and molecules (Fig 2).

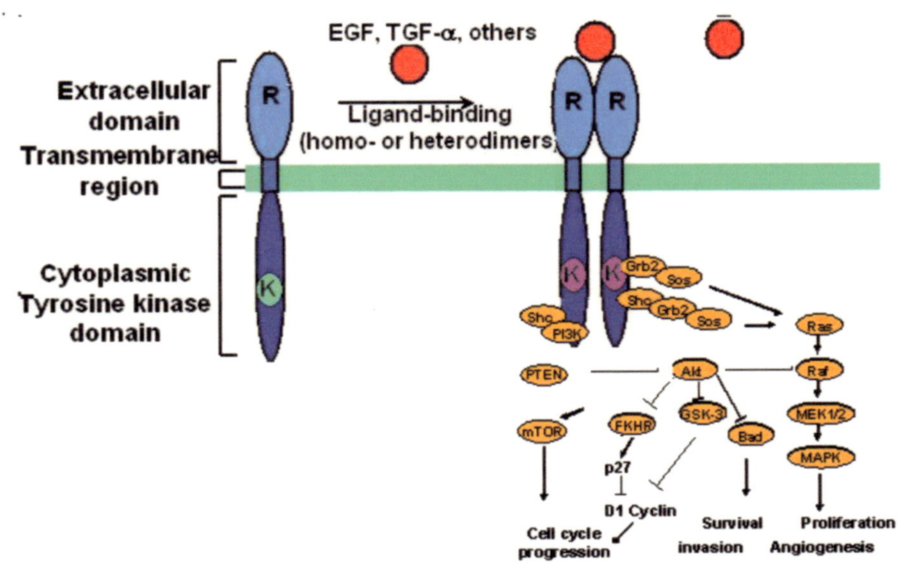

Figure 1. The binding of specific ligands to the receptor activates EGFR and generates a signal transduction cascade through its 2-way main PI3K/Akt and Ras / Raf / MAPK eventually stimulate proliferation, cell cycle progression, repair, angiogenesis and invasion.

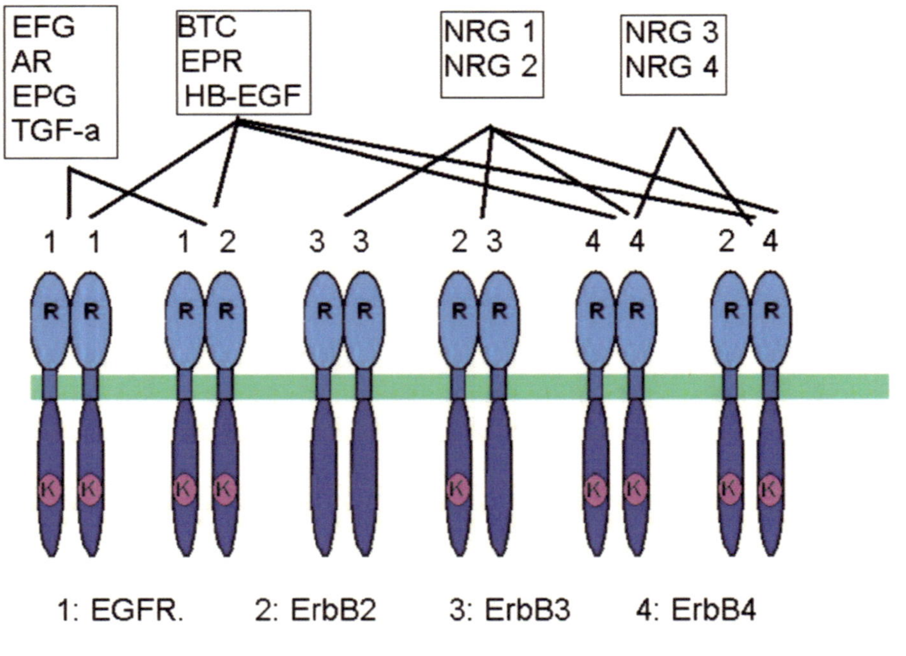

Figure 2. Binding specificities of EGF-related peptide growth factors

Although EGFR plays an important role in maintaining normal cell function, deregulation of EGFR pathway contributes to the development of malignancy progression, inhibition of apoptosis, induction of angiogenesis, promotion of tumor-cell motility and metastasis. Aberrant regulation of the activity or action of EGFR and other members of the RTK family have been involved in multiple cancers, including of brain, lung, breast and ovary. Furthermore, in many tumors EGF-related growth factors are produced either by the tumor cells themselves or are available from surrounding stromal cells, leading to constitutive EGFR activation. In gliomas, EGFR amplification is often accompanied by structural rearrangements that cause in-frame deletions in the extracellular domain of the receptor, the most frequent is the EGFRvIII variant. Somatic mutations in the tyrosine-kinase domain of EGFR were also identified in NSCLC.

When mutated, EGFR tyrosine kinase is constitutively activated, resulting in uncontrolled proliferation, invasion and metastasis. Expression of EGFR and their ligands, especially TGFα, by lung cancer cells, indicates the presence of an autocrine (self-stimulatory) growth factor loop. Activating EGFR mutations are observed in approximately 10% of North American and European populations and 30% to 50% of Asian populations [50] and are significantly more common in never-smokers (100 or less cigarettes per lifetime) or light former smokers (quit 1 year or more ago and less than ten-pack per year smoking history). The leucine to arginine substitution at position 858 (L858R) in exon 21 and short in-frame deletions in exon 19 are the most common mutations seen in adenocarcinomas of the lung. These mutations result in prolonged activation of the receptor and downstream signaling through phosphorylated Akt, in the absence of ligand stimulation of the extracellular domain. EGFR mutations are both prognostic for response rate to chemotherapy and survival irrespective of therapy and are predictive of response to specific inhibitors of the EGFR tyrosine kinase.

4.2. PDGF

Platelet-derived growth factor (PDGF) is a major mitogen for fibroblasts, smooth muscle cells (SMCs), and glia cells. Originally, was identified as a constituent of whole blood serum that was absent in cell-free plasma-derived serum, and was subsequently purified from human platelets [51]. Although the α-granules of platelets are a major storage site for PDGF, can be synthesized by a number of different cell types including fibroblasts, muscle, bone / cartilage, and connective tissue cells.

The synthesis is often increased in response to external stimuli, such as exposure to low oxygen tension, thrombin, or stimulation with various growth factors and cytokines [52].

PDGF is a family of cationic homo- and heterodimers of disulphide-bonded polypeptide chains. In mammals, a total of four different genes encode four PDGF chains (PDGF-A, PDGF-B, PDGF-C, and PDGF-D), which are assembled in five different isoforms known as: AA, AB, BB, CC and DD [53]. All members carry a growth factor core domain containing a conserved set of cysteine residues. The core domain is necessary and sufficient for receptor binding and activation. Classification into PDGFs is based on receptor binding. It has been generally assumed that PDGF is selective for their owns receptors.

PDGF isoforms exert their effects on target cells by activating two structurally related protein tyrosine kinase receptors. The α and β receptors have molecular sizes of 170 and 180 kda, respectively, after maturation of their carbohydrates. Extracellularly, each receptor contains five immunoglobulin-like domains, and intracellularly there is a tyrosine kinase domain that contains a characteristic inserted sequence without homology to kinases.

The human α-receptor gene is localized on chromosome 4q12, close to the genes for the SCF (stem cell factor) receptor and VEGF receptor-2, and the β-receptor gene is on chromosome 5 close to the *CSF*-1 (colony stimulating factor-1) receptor gene [54].

Because PDGF isoforms are dimeric molecules, they bind two receptors simultaneously and dimerize receptors upon binding. The α receptor binds both the A and B chains of PDGF with high affinity, whereas the β receptor binds only the B chain with high affinity. Therefore, PDGF-AA induces $\alpha\alpha$ receptor homodimers, PDGF-AB $\alpha\alpha$ receptor homodimers or $\alpha\beta$ receptor heterodimers, and PDGF-BB all three dimeric combinations of α and β receptors (Fig 3). General mesenchymal expression of PDGFRs is low in vivo, but increases dramatically during inflammation and in culture. Several factors induce PDGFR expression, including TGF-β, estrogen (probably linked to hypertrophic smooth muscle responses in the pregnant uterus), interleukin-1α (IL-1α), basic fibroblast growth factor-2 (FGF-2), tumor necrosis factor-β, and lipopolysaccharide [55].

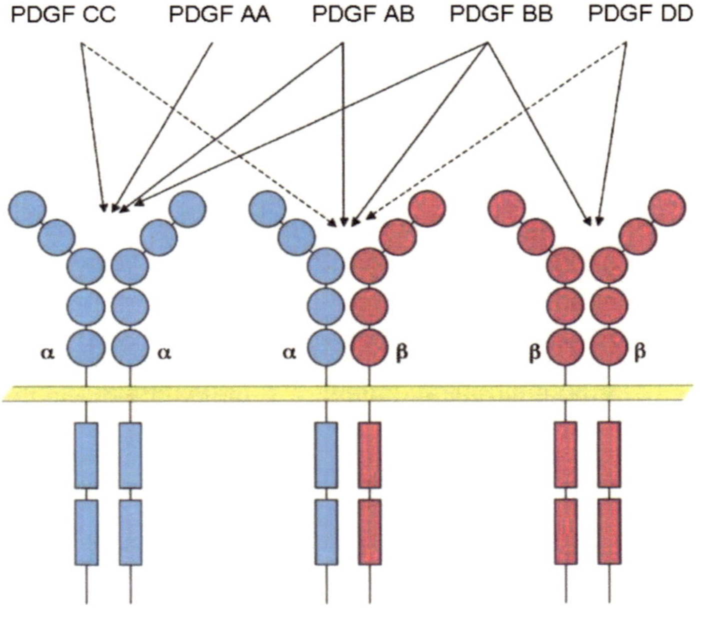

Figure 3. adapted from J Andrae 2008): PDGF–PDGFR interactions. Each chain of the PDGF dimer interacts with one receptor subunit. The active receptor configuration is therefore determined by the ligand dimer configuration. The top panel shows the interactions that have been demonstrated in cell culture. Hatched arrows indicate weak interactions or conflicting results.

The detailed expression patterns of the individual PDGF ligands and receptors are complex. There are some general patterns, however: PDGF-B is mainly expressed in vascular endothelial cells, megakaryocytes, and neurons. PDGF-A and PDGF-C are expressed in epithelial cells, muscle, and neuronal progenitors. PDGF-D expression is less well characterized, but it has been observed in fibroblasts and SMCs at certain locations (possibly suggesting autocrine functions via PDGFR-β). PDGFR-α is expressed in mesenchymal cells. Particularly strong expression of PDGFR-α has been noticed in subtypes of mesenchymal progenitors in lung, skin, and intestine and in oligodendrocyte progenitors (OPs). PDGFR-β is expressed in mesenchyme, particularly in vascular SMCs (vSMCs) and pericytes.

PDGF biosynthesis and processing are controlled at multiple levels and differ for the different PDGFs. PDGF-A and PDGF-B become disulphide-linked into dimers already as propeptides. PDGF-C and PDGF-D have been less studied on this regard. PDGF-A and PDGF-B contain N-terminal pro-domains that are removed intracellularly by furin or related proprotein convertases. Likely, PDGF-B also requires N-terminal propeptide removal to become active. In contrast, PDGF-C and PDGF-D are not processed intracellularly but are instead secreted as latent (conditionally inactive) ligands. Activation in the extracellular space requires dissociation of the growth factor domain.

Dimerization is the key event in PDGF receptor activation as it allows for receptor autophosphorylation on tyrosine residues in the intracellular domain. Autophosphorylation activates the receptor kinase and provides docking sites for downstream signaling molecules and further signal propagation involves protein–protein interactions through specific domains; e.g., Src homology 2 (SH2) and phosphotyrosine binding (PTB) domains recognizing phosphorylated tyrosines, SH3 domains recognizing proline-rich regions, pleckstrin homology (PH) domains recognizing membrane phospholipids, and PDZ domains recognizing C terminal specific sequences. Most of the PDGFR effectors bind to specific sites on the phosphorylated receptors through their SH2 domains. Both PDGFR-α and PDGFR-β engage several well-characterized signaling pathways, e.g. Ras-MAPK, PI3K and PLC-γ, which are known to be involved in multiple cellular and developmental responses [56].

The PDGFR is expressed on capillary endothelial cells and PDGF has been shown to have an angiogenic effect. The effect is, however, weaker than that of fibroblast growth factors or VEGF, and PDGF does not appear to be of importance for the initial formation of blood vessels. PDGF B-chain produced by capillaries may have an important role to recruit pericytes that is likely to be required to promote the structural integrity of the vessels. PDGF has also been implicated in the regulation of the tonus of blood vessels [57].

PDGF functions have been implicated in a broad range of diseases. For a few of them, i.e., some cancers, there is a strong evidence for a causative role of PDGF signaling in this human disease process. In these cases, genetic aberrations cause uncontrolled PDGF signaling in the tumor cells.

4.3. VEG/PF

Vascular endothelial growth/permeability factor (VEG/PF) is a 40 kda disulphide-linked dimeric glycoprotein that is active in increasing blood vessel permeability, endothelial cell growth and angiogenesis. These properties suggest that the expression of VEG/PF by tumor cells could contribute to the increased neovascularization and vessel permeability that are associated with tumor vasculature. The cDNA sequence of VEG/PF from human U937 cells was shown to code for a 189-amino acid polypeptide that is similar in structure to the B chain of PDGF-B and other PDGF-B-related proteins. The overall identity with PDGF-B is 18%. However, all eight of the cysteines in PDGF-B were conserved in human VEG/PF, an indication that the folding of the two proteins is probably similar. Clusters of basic amino acids in the COOH-terminal halves of human VEG/PF and PDGF-B are also prevalent. Thus, VEG/PF appears to be related to the PDGF/v-sis family of proteins [58].

5. Angiogenesis and radiological assessment techniques

Neoangiogenesis, the formation of new blood vessels from a pre-existing vascular network, is essential for tumor growth, tumor proliferation and metastasis. The angiogenesis process is regulated by different proangiogenic and antiangiogenic factors, being the primary stimulus of new vessel formation the hypoxia induced by expansion of the growing tumor mass [59].

Tumor angiogenesis is an attractive target for anticancer therapy, and a wide range of novel therapies directed against tumor vascularity has been developed. Because many antiangiogenic agents are not cytotoxic but instead produce disease stabilization, measurement of tumor size alone may be not informative regarding therapeutic effects. For that reason, there has been great interest in the use of physiologic, rather than solely anatomic, imaging techniques [60]. Tumor vascularity has different features that are characteristic of malignancy, such as spatial heterogeneity, chaotic structure, fragility and high permeability to macromolecules. These structural abnormalities of new tumor vessels lead to pathophysiologic changes within the neoplastic tissue, including an increase in capillary permeability, volume of extravascular-extracellular space, and tumor perfusion, that permit distinction of malignant from benign vascularity with functional imaging techniques.

Several commonly available imaging modalities, including magnetic resonance (MR), computed tomography (CT), ultrasound and positron emission tomography (PET), have been used to indirectly assess the angiogenic status of human tumors [61]. But perfusion imaging with MR, and specially CT, are the most useful in clinical practice. They have the advantage of good spatial resolution, minimal invasiveness and rapid acquisition of data. Both techniques sequentially demonstrate passage of a bolus of contrast medium through a region of interest and allow quantification of the profile of tissue enhancement.

http://dx.doi.org/10.5772/54309

6. Perfusion CT

The fundamental principle of perfusion CT is based on the temporal changes in tissue attenuation after intravenous administration of iodinated contrast material (CM). This enhancement depends on the tissue iodine concentration, existing a direct linear relationship between contrast concentration and CT enhancement [62].

Recent progress in multidetector CT technology has enabled the rapid scanning of large anatomic volumes with high resolution. In perfusion CT, repeated series of images of the volume analyzed are performed in quick succession before, during and after intravenous administration of CM. The ensuing tissue enhancement can be divided into two phases based on CM distribution: a initial phase where the enhancement is attributable to the distribution of contrast within the intravascular space ("first pass", lasting 40-60 secs. from the contrast arrival), and a second phase as contrast diffuses from the intravascular to the extravascular compartment across the capillary basement membrane (2-5 minutes duration). To objectively quantify the "real" perfusion parameters of tissues from the density difference produced by the contribution of contrast material, a mathematic model is applied to the dynamic CT data. The quantitative parameters generated include blood volume (BV), blood flow (BF), mean transit time and capillary permeability surface.

Perfusion CT is a biomarker for angiogenesis that have been validated with other surrogate markers, such as VEGF levels, tumor perfusion and microvascular density (Fig 4) [63]. There has been a gradual increase of its use in oncology, ranging the wide spectrum of clinical applications of this technique, from lesion characterization, (differentiation between benign and malignant lesions), to prognostic information based on tumor vascularity and monitoring therapeutic effects of chemoradiation and antiangiogenic drugs. In a recent study using a 320-detector row CT, Ohno et al. concluded that perfusion CT has the potential to be more specific and accurate than PET/CT for differentiating malignant from benign pulmonary nodules [64]. Another study have also shown that in patients with NSCLC treated with sorafenib and erlotinib, early changes in tumor blood flow were predictive of objective response and tended to indicate a longer progression-free survival [65].

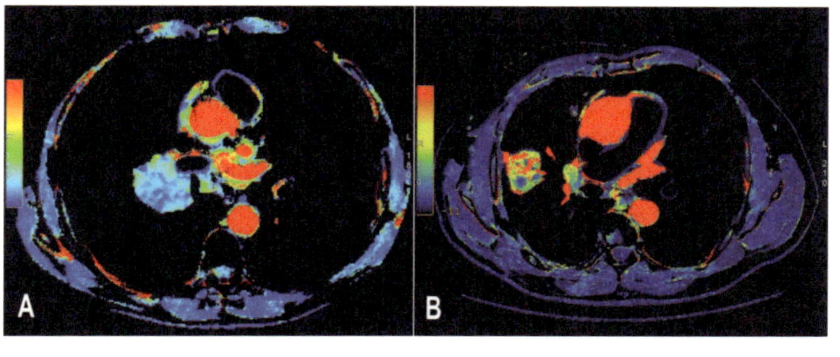

Figure 4. Parametric maps of perfusion CT studies representing blood flow in two different patients with NSCLC. (A) Tumor with very low perfusion depicted in blue and (B) a highly vascularized neoplasm showing yellow and red zones (scale at left).

Radiation exposure, the requirement of long breath holding during chest imaging acquisition and lack of standardized protocols, remain potential drawbacks of this technique. However, implementation of low-dose scanning strategies may allow a more widespread use in the future.

7. Dynamic MR

Quantification of tumor vascularity by dynamic MR (DCE MR) is technically more challenging than perfusion CT because there is a lack of a direct relationship between MR signal intensity and contrast agent concentration. This is due to the fact that tissue signal intensity on MR is related to the effect of CM on water in the microenvironment, which changes tissue relaxivity in complex and unpredictable ways [66].

While perfusion CT yield information is based predominantly on the first pass of CM (BV, BF), the MR imaging technique may sample a volume of interest over a longer time and yields parameters that reflect microvessel perfusion, permeability and extracellular leakage of space. In addition, by applying pharmacokinetic models to the MR imaging acquisitions, it is possible to calculate quantitative parameters, such as the transfer constant (K^{trans}) that describes the transendothelial transport of the CM.

A central flaw of dynamic MR is that acquisition and pharmacokinetic models vary widely. Thus, comparing studies from different institutions is difficult. This technique, on the other hand, is of limited value in organs with physiological movement such as the lungs.

Few studies have applied dynamic MR in the assessment of lung cancer. Ohno et al [67] evaluated the role of DCE MR as a prognostic indicator in NSCLC patients treated with chemotherapy using cisplatin and vincristine. In their study, the mean survival period of patients with lower slope of enhancement was significantly longer than that seen in the group with higher slope of enhancement. This study provides promising data for the application of dynamic MR in response assessment to chemotherapy and targeted therapy.

8. Current state of antiangiogenic therapy for NSCLC: VEGF as target treatment

In this section, we analyze the activity of a monoclonal antibody (bevacizumab) and other new antiangiogenic therapies.

8.1. Bevacizumab

Bevacizumab is a monoclonal antibody directed against VEGF and was the first antiangiogenic drug approved for the treatment of advanced NSCLC. Currently it's the only approved in this setting in Europe and the USA.

After proving the improvement in the response rate (RR) and progression free survival (PFS) of bevacizumab together with chemotherapy in first line in a randomized phase II study in which 99 patients with advanced or metastatic NSCLC were included [68], the ECOG group undertook a phase III trial (ECOG 4599) in first line, in which patients with brain metastasis, hemoptysis, and squamous histology were excluded, due to the risk of hemoptysis observed in the previous study with this histology [69]. The studied randomized 878 patients with recurrent or advanced NSCLC to receive carboplatin/paclitaxel with or without bevacizumab on a dose of 15 mg/kg every 21 days and crossover was not allowed. The main objective, overall survival (OS), was improved in the trial arm: 12.3 months vs 10.3 months, with a hazard ratio (HR): 0.79 (95% CI: 0.67-0.92; p=0.003). In addition, the RR was also improved (35 vs 15% (p<0.001)) and the PFS went from 4.5 to 6.2 months (HR: 0.66; 95% CI: 0.57-0-77, p<0.001). However, adding bevacizumab to the chemotherapy also increased toxicity; there were 15 toxic deaths (2 in the arm of chemotherapy alone) due to pulmonary hemorrhage, digestive bleeding, febrile neutropenia, ictus and lung embolism. A subgroup analysis found that patients over 70 had a higher incidence of grade 3-5 toxicities (87 vs 61%).

The AVAiL study [70] randomized 1043 patients to receive cisplatin and gemcitabine with or without bevacizumab in a dose of 7.5 or 15 mg/kg each 21 days. In this study the main goal was PFS, which was higher in patients which received the drug than those who took placebo, both in small dose arm (6.7 months vs 6.1 months; HR: 0.75, p=0.003) as well as in higher one (6.5 months vs 6.1 months, HR: 0.82, p=0.03). Nevertheless, OS didn't improve, which could be explained by the high percentage of patients who received treatment afterwards (more than 60%). Regarding toxicity, 7 patients died due to lung hemorrhage in the trial arm (2 in the control trial), although it was observed that in patients who were under anticoagulant treatment there was no lung hemorrhage.

The SAiL safety study, which included more than 2000 patients, showed the effectiveness of combining other doublets of chemotherapy; in terms of safety it displayed a grade 3 or higher lung hemorrhage incidence only in 1% of the patients [71].

An efficiency meta-analysis published in 2011 confirms effectiveness in terms of PFS, presenting uncertainty in terms of improvement of OS [72].

A meta-analysis published recently with 2210 patients evaluated the bevacizumab toxicity profile with high dose of bevacizumab (15 mg/kg), and stated that bevacizumab is related to a higher risk of toxicity deaths (HR: 2.04; 95% CI: 1.18-3.52), but it was not the case in lower doses of 7.5 mg/kg (HR: 1.20; 95% CI: 0.60-2.41). In addition, bevacizumab was associated to a greater incidence of grade 3-4 toxicities, especially in the group of high doses [73].

More studies have been conducted in sub-populations, for example, the PASSPORT study in 109 patients with brain metastasis, subgroup that had not been included in previous studies, and which proved that bevacizumab can be administrated in patients with controlled brain metastasis [74]. Another review on the incidence of bleeding in patients with brain metastasis treated with antiangiogenic drugs proved to be safe when it is administered to treated patients as well as patients with metastasis that appears during treatment [75].

The combination of bevacizumab with some of the new agents has been studied as well. In the ATLAS study, after having received four cycles of cisplatin-based chemotherapy and bevacizumab, patients were randomized to receive treatment with bevacizumab (15 mg/kg) and erlotinib (150 mg daily) or only bevacizumab. The main objective of this study was reached (PFS), with 4.8 months vs 3.7 months (HR: 0.72, p=0.0012); nevertheless no improvement was made in OS, a secondary goal of the study (14.4 months vs 13.3 months; p=0.56) [76].

The phase III BeTa trial compared the activity of the combination of bevacizumab and erlotinib vs erlotinib in second line in 636 patients. An improvement in PFS was found (3.4 vs 1.7 months; HR: 0.62, p<0.0001), but again, no significant differences were found in OS (9.3 vs 9.2 months; p=0.75)

Hypertension has been found to be a marker of clinical benefit from bevacizumab in various malignancies [77], although no single biomarker have proven to be ready for clinical use. Cytokines and angiogenic factors profiling may help identify drug-specific markers of activity.

8.2. Aflibercept

Aflibercept (VEGF-Trap) is a recombining fusion protein, which is added to VEGFR-1, VEGFR-2 and to the placental growth factor (PlGF).

In a phase II trial in patients with lung adenocarcinoma treated after several treatment lines, aflibercept in a dose of 4 mg/kg was administered intravenously every 14 days, reaching a RR of 2%, with a PFS of 2.7 months and an OS of 6.2 months [78]. A phase III trial in second line after failure to cisplatin-based chemotherapy compared aflibercept vs docetaxel (VITAL trial). This trial showed an improved RR (23.3& vs 8.9%) and PFS (HR: 0.82), but the primary endpoint, OS, was not reached (HR: 1.01).

9. Vascular disrupting agents

Vadimezan, fosbretabulin and plinabulin are vascular disrupting agents (VDA); fosbretabulin selectively disrupts VE-cadherin and plinabulin acts on cytoskeleton. A phase II trial of carboplatin, paclitaxel, bevacizumab and fosbretabulin was well tolerated and with a trend to improve OS and PFS [79], also a phase II trial with docetaxel with or without plinabulin showed a higher response rate with the combination (55% vs 5%) [80]; however, a randomized phase III study with vadimezan in first line failed to show an improvement in OS [81].

10. Multi-targeted tyrosine kinase inhibitors

Several anti-angiogenic small-molecule tyrosine kinase inhibitors (TKIs) are in current clinical development. An advantage of TKIs includes the fact that they inhibit multiple receptors simultaneously, with anti-angiogenic and anti-proliferative activity against NSCLC, thereby potentially providing a higher likelihood of single-agent activity. Another benefit is that these agents are often available orally, offering patients greater convenience. However, toxicity remains a concern given the multi-targeted kinase inhibition and the additive adverse effects that may be of particular concern when the agents are combined with chemotherapy.

11. Sorafenib

Sorafenib is an oral multi-kinase inhibitor of VEGFR-2 and -3, PDGFR-β, RAF-kinase, c-Kit, RET, and Ftl-3.

In the phase II ECOG 2501 trial, 342 patients with NSCLC who has failed at least two prior chemotherapy regimens received sorafenib for two cycles. Those patients who were noted to have stable disease after two cycles (n = 97) were randomized to receive sorafenib or placebo. Sorafenib prolonged PFS compared with placebo (3.6 versus 1.9 months) [82]. In another phase II trial, of 52 patients with relapsed or refractory advanced NSCLC, 59% achieved SD, and in these patients, median PFS was 5.5 months [83].

The results of two phase III trials in the first-line treatment of NSCLC, ESCAPE (sorafenib plus paclitaxel/carboplatin) and NEXUS (sorafenib plus gemcitabine/cisplatin), were unsatisfactory. Because of the safety findings from the ESCAPE trial, patients with squamous cell histology were withdrawn from the NEXUS trial in February 2008 and excluded from analysis. Median OS, the primary endpoint of both trials, was similar in the sorafenib and placebo groups [84,85].

The Biomarker-Integrated Approaches of Targeted Therapy for Lung Cancer Elimination (BATTLE) study randomized pretreated lung cancer patients to erlotinib, vandetanib, erlotinib plus bexarotene or sorafenib based upon biomarker results obtained from individual patients. K-ras-mutant patients treated with sorafenib had a non-statistically significant trend toward improved disease control rate (DCR) (61 versus 32%, p = 0.11), suggesting a preferential benefit of sorafenib in k-ras-mutant patients [86].

Phase III MISSION trial of sorafenib in patients with advanced relapsed or refractory non-squamous NSCLC whose disease progressed after two or three previous treatments, did not meet its primary endpoint of improving OS. An improvement in the secondary endpoint of PFS was observed [87].

These findings have led to suspend the development of sorafenib in NSCLC.

12. Vandetanib

Vandetanib is an oral TKI that inhibits VEGFR-2 and -3, RET and EGFR.

Vandetanib in combination with carboplatin/paclitaxel resulted in prolonged PFS (56 weeks; HR= 0.76, p= 0.098) compared with carboplatin/paclitaxel alone (52 weeks) in previously untreated patients with advanced NSCLC. The secondary endpoint of OS was not significantly different between the two arms [88]. Another phase II trial showed that vandetanib in combination with docetaxel was superior to docetaxel alone in pretreated NSCLC patients with regard to PFS (18.7 weeks versus 12 weeks; HR = 0.64, p = 0.037) [89].

The phase III ZODIAC trial randomized patients with advanced NSCLC to receive either docetaxel/vandetanib or docetaxel/placebo as second-line treatment. Although vandetanib improved ORR (17 versus 10%, p= 0.0001) and PFS (HR: 0.79, p< 0.0001), OS was not significantly improved (HR: 0.91, p= 0.196) [90]. In the ZEAL trial, vandetanib was investigated in combination with pemetrexed also in the second-line setting. Despite an improvement in ORR (19 versus 8%, p < 0.001), this study did not meet its primary endpoint of PFS (HR: 0.86, p = 0.108) [91]. In another phase III trial (ZEPHYR), patients who had progressed after chemotherapy and erlotinib were randomized to vandetanib versus placebo. PFS was improved (HR: 0.63, p < 0.0001), but not OS (HR: 0.95, p = 0.527) [92]. The above phase III trials did not carry out stratified analysis on the EGFR gene status and therefore were not able to further identify the potential populations that may benefit from vandetanib.

These results led to withdrawal of the application for approval of vandetanib in NSCLC.

13. Sunitinib

Sunitinib is an oral TKI of VEGFR-1, -2, -3, PDGFR-α/β, c-kit, Flt-3 and RET.

It has been studied in advanced NSCLC in two phase II trials. In the first one, 63 pretreated patients received sunitinib as single agent, achieving an ORR of 11.1% (95%CI: 4.6–21.6), median PFS of 12 weeks (95%CI: 10.0-16.1) and median OS of 23.4 weeks (95%CI: 17.0-28.3) [93]. In the other phase II trial, 47 pretreated patients received sunitinib on a continuous-dosing schedule (37.5 mg/day). The ORR was only 2.1%, but median PFS and OS were 11.9 weeks (95%CI: 8.6-14.1) and 37.1 weeks (95%CI: 31.1-69.7), respectively [94].

There are ongoing studies investigating sunitinib in patients with NSCLC, including the phase II CALGB 30704 trial evaluating sunitinib as second-line therapy and the phase III CALGB 30607 study of sunitinib as maintenance therapy.

14. Other multi-targeted TKIs

Axitinib, with VEGFR, PDGFR-β and c-Kit as its main targets, is currently the most potent TKI in inhibiting VEGFR signal pathways. In a phase II study in advanced NSCLC, in which 28% of patients had received no prior chemotherapy, ORR was 9.4%, with PFS and OS of 4.9 and 14.8 months, respectively [95]. Currently, three ongoing phase II studies are exploring the effectiveness and safety of axitinib-based combination therapies in non-squamous (AGILE1030: with paclitaxel/carboplatin; AGILE1039: with pemetrexed/cisplatin) and squamous NSCLC (AGILE1038: with cisplatin/gemcitabine).

Motesanib mainly inhibits targets including VEGFR, PDGFR, c-Kit and RET. In a phase II study of motesanib or bevacizumab in combination with carboplatin/paclitaxel as frontline treatment for advanced non-squamous NSCLC, the efficacy was similar, with a median PFS of 7.7 months (versus 8.3 months with bevacizumab) and a median OS of 14.0 months in both arms [96]. However, the phase III study of motesanib plus carboplatin/paclitaxel in patients with non-squamous advanced NSCLC (MONET1) did not meet its primary endpoint of improved OS (HR: 0.89, p = 0.137) [97].

BIBF 1120 inhibits VEGFR-1, -2 and -3, in addition to PDGFR-α/β and FGFR-1-3. In a phase II trial of 73 patients with relapsed or advanced NSCLC, the median PFS and OS were 11.6 and 37.7 weeks, respectively, with a disease control rate (DCR) of 46% [98]. BIBF 1120 is being studied, in the second-line NSCLC setting, in two phase III trials, in combination with docetaxel (LUME-Lung 1) and with pemetrexed (LUME-Lung 2).

A phase Ib/II study of cabozantinib, a TKI with potent activity against MET, VEGFR-2, RET, c-Kit and Ftl-3, with or without erlotinib in pretreated advanced NSCLC patients showed that the combination was well tolerated with evidence of clinical activity in a largely erlotinib pretreated cohort, including patients with EGFR T790M mutation and MET amplification [99].

Another multikinase inhibitors like pazopanib are in an earlier stage of development.

Although multitargeted TKIs have made certain advances in treating NSCLC, the outcomes remain unsatisfactory if they were applied non-selectively among NSCLC patients. Among the non-selective populations, TKI monotherapies showed no significant differences when compared with mono-targeted agent therapies (erlotinib, gefitinib) in treating NSCLC in terms of ORR, PFS and OS. Therefore, it is extremely important to identify populations that are suitable for TKIs. The future of multi-targeted drugs is highly depended on the capability of delivering these molecule-targeted therapies to patients most likely to benefit.

15. Conclusions

In recent years, we have acquired a lot of information regarding the role of angiogenesis and its pathophysiological relationship with some types of neoplasias, engaging in processes such as tumour growth and dissemination capacity as loco-regional as distant. In lung cancer, we know that neoangiogenesis is the result of the action of several growth factors (mainly VEGF, TGF-alpha, EGF, VEG/PF and PDGF) whose output is controlled by transcription factors hypoxia-induced such as HIF-1, whose expression has been associated as an independent factor of poor prognosis. Acquired knowledge has allowed designing therapeutic strategies aimed at blocking the action of various pro-angiogenic factors and thereby altering the disease natural course. Some drugs acting against VEGF, as bevacizumab, have demonstrated clinical efficacy improving OS and PFS although with treatment-related toxicities expected with blocking this pathway, as showed some trials, particularly in patients subsets with a known clinical profile that when is present makes it more susceptible to those complications. Another line of research has been that of small-molecule tyrosine kinase inhibitors (sorafenib, vandetanib, sunitinib, axitinib, pazopanib and motesanib), showing some benefits in PFS but without a positive impact in OS when were applied non-selectively among NSCLC patients, so in the future probably we will need identify populations with a right profile that allows us to predict who have more chance to benefit from this therapy. Structural abnormalities in tumor neovascularization lead to pathophysiological changes within the neoplastic tissue. The study of these functional changes have allowed to develop imaging techniques that, not only differentiate a benign lesion from other malignant, but also provide prognostic information and monitor the therapeutic effects of drugs used. Thus, techniques such as perfusion CT and dynamic MR allow anatomical and functional assessment of neoplasia, based on the characteristics and changes of intratumoral capillary network.

Author details

S. Vázquez[1], U. Anido[2], M. Lázaro[3], L. Santomé[4], J. Afonso[5], O. Fernández[6], A. Martínez de Alegría[2] and L. A. Aparicio[7*]

*Address all correspondence to: Luis.M.Anton.Aparicio@sergas.es.

1 Hospital Universitario Lucus Augusti, Lugo, Spain

2 Complexo Hospitalario Universitario de Santiago, Santiago de Compostela, Spain

3 Complexo Hospitalario Universitario de Vigo, Vigo, Spain

4 POVISA, Vigo, Spain

5 Hospital Arquitecto Marcide, Ferrol, Spain

6 Complexo Hospitalario Universitario de Ourense, Ourense, Spain

7 Complexo Hospitalario Universitario de A Coruña, A Coruña, Spain

References

[1] Folkman J. What is the evidence that tumors are angiogenesis dependent? J Natl Cancer Inst 1990;82(1):4-6.

[2] Carmeliet P, Jain RK. Angiogenesis in cancer and other diseases. Nature 2000, Sep 14;407(6801):249-57.

[3] Jain RK. Molecular regulation of vessel maturation. Nat Med 2003, Jun;9(6):685-93.

[4] Gerber HP, Kowalski J, Sherman D, Eberhard DA, Ferrara N. Complete inhibition of rhabdomyosarcoma xenograft growth and neovascularization requires blockade of both tumor and host vascular endothelial growth factor. Cancer Res 2000, Nov 15;60(22):6253-8.

[5] Hanahan D, Folkman J. Patterns and emerging mechanisms of the angiogenic switch during tumorigenesis. Cell 1996, Aug 9;86(3):353-64.

[6] Kaelin WG. The von hippel-lindau protein, HIF hydroxylation, and oxygen sensing. Biochem Biophys Res Commun 2005, Dec 9;338(1):627-38.

[7] Imoto H, Osaki T, Taga S, Ohgami A, Ichiyoshi Y, Yasumoto K. Vascular endothelial growth factor expression in non-small-cell lung cancer: Prognostic significance in squamous cell carcinoma. J Thorac Cardiovasc Surg 1998, May;115(5):1007-14.

[8] Herbst RS, Fidler IJ. Angiogenesis and lung cancer: Potential for therapy. Clin Cancer Res 2000, Dec;6(12):4604-6.

[9] Cox G, Jones JL, Walker RA, Steward WP, O'Byrne KJ. Angiogenesis and non-small cell lung cancer. Lung Cancer 2000, Feb;27(2):81-100.

[10] Tamura M, Ohta Y, Kajita T, Kimura K, Go T, Oda M, et al. Plasma VEGF concentration can predict the tumor angiogenic capacity in non-small cell lung cancer. Oncol Rep 2001;8(5):1097-102.

[11] Takigawa N, Segawa Y, Fujimoto N, Hotta K, Eguchi K. Elevated vascular endothelial growth factor levels in sera of patients with lung cancer. Anticancer Res 1998;18(2B):1251-4.

[12] Linder C, Linder S, Munck-Wikland E, Strander H. Independent expression of serum vascular endothelial growth factor (VEGF) and basic fibroblast growth factor (bfgf) in patients with carcinoma and sarcoma. Anticancer Res 1998;18(3B):2063-8.

[13] Matsuyama W, Hashiguchi T, Mizoguchi A, Iwami F, Kawabata M, Arimura K, Osame M. Serum levels of vascular endothelial growth factor dependent on the stage progression of lung cancer. Chest 2000, Oct;118(4):948-51.

[14] Choi JH, Kim HC, Lim HY, Nam DK, Kim HS, Yi JW, et al. Vascular endothelial growth factor in the serum of patients with non-small cell lung cancer: Correlation with platelet and leukocyte counts. Lung Cancer 2001;33(2-3):171-9.

[15] Laack E, Köhler A, Kugler C, Dierlamm T, Knuffmann C, Vohwinkel G, et al. Pretreatment serum levels of matrix metalloproteinase-9 and vascular endothelial growth factor in non-small-cell lung cancer. Ann Oncol 2002, Oct;13(10):1550-7.

[16] Jäger R, List B, Knabbe C, Souttou B, Raulais D, Zeiler T, et al. Serum levels of the angiogenic factor pleiotrophin in relation to disease stage in lung cancer patients. Br J Cancer 2002, Mar 18;86(6):858-63.

[17] Suzuki M, Iizasa T, Ko E, Baba M, Saitoh Y, Shibuya K, et al. Serum endostatin correlates with progression and prognosis of non-small cell lung cancer. Lung Cancer 2002, Jan;35(1):29-34.

[18] Brattström D, Bergqvist M, Hesselius P, Larsson A, Lamberg K, Wernlund J, et al. Elevated preoperative serum levels of angiogenic cytokines correlate to larger primary tumours and poorer survival in non-small cell lung cancer patients. Lung Cancer 2002, Jul;37(1):57-63.

[19] Folkman J. Antiangiogenesis agents. In: DeVita VT, Lawrence TS, Rosenberg SA, editors. Principles & Practice of Oncology. Lippincott Williams & Wilkins; 2011.

[20] Carter SK. Clinical strategy for the development of angiogenesis inhibitors. Oncologist 2000;5 Suppl 1:51-4.

[21] Semenza GL, Wang GL. A nuclear factor induced by hypoxia via de novo protein synthesis binds to the human erythropoietin gene enhancer at a site required for transcriptional activation. Mol Cell Biol 1992, Dec;12(12):5447-54.

[22] Swinson DE, Jones JL, Cox G, Richardson D, Harris AL, O'Byrne KJ. Hypoxia-inducible factor-1 alpha in non small cell lung cancer: Relation to growth factor, protease and apoptosis pathways. Int J Cancer 2004, Aug 10;111(1):43-50.

[23] Iliopoulos O, Levy AP, Jiang C, Kaelin WG, Goldberg MA. Negative regulation of hypoxia-inducible genes by the von hippel-lindau protein. Proc Natl Acad Sci U S A 1996, Oct 1;93(20):10595-9.

[24] Maxwell PH, Wiesener MS, Chang GW, Clifford SC, Vaux EC, Cockman ME, et al. The tumour suppressor protein VHL targets hypoxia-inducible factors for oxygen-dependent proteolysis. Nature 1999, May 20;399(6733):271-5.

[25] Ferrara N, Gerber HP, LeCouter J. The biology of VEGF and its receptors. Nat Med 2003, Jun;9(6):669-76.

[26] Mizukami Y, Kohgo Y, Chung DC. Hypoxia inducible factor-1 independent pathways in tumor angiogenesis. Clin Cancer Res 2007, Oct 1;13(19):5670-4.

[27] Wykoff CC, Beasley NJ, Watson PH, Turner KJ, Pastorek J, Sibtain A, et al. Hypoxia-inducible expression of tumor-associated carbonic anhydrases. Cancer Res 2000, Dec 15;60(24):7075-83.

[28] Beasley NJ, Wykoff CC, Watson PH, Leek R, Turley H, Gatter K, et al. Carbonic anhydrase IX, an endogenous hypoxia marker, expression in head and neck squamous cell carcinoma and its relationship to hypoxia, necrosis, and microvessel density. Cancer Res 2001, Jul 1;61(13):5262-7.

[29] Loncaster JA, Harris AL, Davidson SE, Logue JP, Hunter RD, Wycoff CC, et al. Carbonic anhydrase (CA IX) expression, a potential new intrinsic marker of hypoxia: Correlations with tumor oxygen measurements and prognosis in locally advanced carcinoma of the cervix. Cancer Res 2001, Sep 1;61(17):6394-9.

[30] Airley R, Loncaster J, Davidson S, Bromley M, Roberts S, Patterson A, et al. Glucose transporter glut-1 expression correlates with tumor hypoxia and predicts metastasis-free survival in advanced carcinoma of the cervix. Clin Cancer Res 2001, Apr;7(4): 928-34.

[31] Swinson DE, Jones JL, Richardson D, Wykoff C, Turley H, Pastorek J, et al. Carbonic anhydrase IX expression, a novel surrogate marker of tumor hypoxia, is associated with a poor prognosis in non-small-cell lung cancer. J Clin Oncol 2003, Feb 1;21(3): 473-82.

[32] Carmeliet P, Dor Y, Herbert JM, Fukumura D, Brusselmans K, Dewerchin M, et al. Role of hif-1alpha in hypoxia-mediated apoptosis, cell proliferation and tumour angiogenesis. Nature 1998, Jul 30;394(6692):485-90.

[33] Stein I, Neeman M, Shweiki D, Itin A, Keshet E. Stabilization of vascular endothelial growth factor mrna by hypoxia and hypoglycemia and coregulation with other ischemia-induced genes. Mol Cell Biol 1995, Oct;15(10):5363-8.

[34] Folkman J. Tumor angiogenesis: Therapeutic implications. N Engl J Med 1971, Nov 18;285(21):1182-6.

[35] Poon RT, Fan ST, Wong J. Clinical implications of circulating angiogenic factors in cancer patients. J Clin Oncol 2001, Feb 15;19(4):1207-25.

[36] Tanno S, Ohsaki Y, Nakanishi K, Toyoshima E, Kikuchi K. Human small cell lung cancer cells express functional VEGF receptors, VEGFR-2 and VEGFR-3. Lung Cancer 2004, Oct;46(1):11-9.

[37] Ludovini V, Gregorc V, Pistola L, Mihaylova Z, Floriani I, Darwish S, et al. Vascular endothelial growth factor, p53, rb, bcl-2 expression and response to chemotherapy in advanced non-small cell lung cancer. Lung Cancer 2004, Oct;46(1):77-85.

[38] Ishii H, Yazawa T, Sato H, Suzuki T, Ikeda M, Hayashi Y, et al. Enhancement of pleural dissemination and lymph node metastasis of intrathoracic lung cancer cells by vascular endothelial growth factors (vegfs). Lung Cancer 2004, Sep;45(3):325-37.

[39] Stefanou D, Batistatou A, Arkoumani E, Ntzani E, Agnantis NJ. Expression of vascular endothelial growth factor (VEGF) and association with microvessel density in small-cell and non-small-cell lung carcinomas. Histol Histopathol 2004, Jan;19(1): 37-42.

[40] Cressey R, Wattananupong O, Lertprasertsuke N, Vinitketkumnuen U. Alteration of protein expression pattern of vascular endothelial growth factor (VEGF) from soluble to cell-associated isoform during tumourigenesis. BMC Cancer 2005;5:128.

[41] Shimanuki Y, Takahashi K, Cui R, Hori S, Takahashi F, Miyamoto H, Fukurchi Y. Role of serum vascular endothelial growth factor in the prediction of angiogenesis and prognosis for non-small cell lung cancer. Lung 2005;183(1):29-42.

[42] Yoshimoto A, Kasahara K, Nishio M, Hourai T, Sone T, Kimura H, et al. Changes in angiogenic growth factor levels after gefitinib treatment in non-small cell lung cancer. Jpn J Clin Oncol 2005, May;35(5):233-8.

[43] Wakeling AE, Guy SP, Woodburn JR, Ashton SE, Curry BJ, Barker AJ, Gibson KH. ZD1839 (iressa): An orally active inhibitor of epidermal growth factor signaling with potential for cancer therapy. Cancer Res 2002, Oct 15;62(20):5749-54.

[44] Ciardiello F, Caputo R, Bianco R, Damiano V, Pomatico G, De Placido S, et al. Antitumor effect and potentiation of cytotoxic drugs activity in human cancer cells by ZD-1839 (iressa), an epidermal growth factor receptor-selective tyrosine kinase inhibitor. Clin Cancer Res 2000, May;6(5):2053-63.

[45] Ciardiello F, Caputo R, Bianco R, Damiano V, Fontanini G, Cuccato S, et al. Inhibition of growth factor production and angiogenesis in human cancer cells by ZD1839 (iressa), a selective epidermal growth factor receptor tyrosine kinase inhibitor. Clin Cancer Res 2001, May;7(5):1459-65.

[46] Hirata A, Ogawa S, Kometani T, Kuwano T, Naito S, Kuwano M, Ono M. ZD1839 (iressa) induces antiangiogenic effects through inhibition of epidermal growth factor receptor tyrosine kinase. Cancer Res 2002, May 1;62(9):2554-60.

[47] Reck M, von Pawel J, Zatloukal P, Ramlau R, Gorbounova V, Hirsh V, et al. Overall survival with cisplatin-gemcitabine and bevacizumab or placebo as first-line therapy for nonsquamous non-small-cell lung cancer: Results from a randomised phase III trial (avail). Ann Oncol 2010, Sep;21(9):1804-9.

[48] Sandler A, Gray R, Perry MC, Brahmer J, Schiller JH, Dowlati A, et al. Paclitaxel-carboplatin alone or with bevacizumab for non-small-cell lung cancer. N Engl J Med 2006, Dec 14;355(24):2542-50.

[49] Citri A, Yarden Y. EGF-ERBB signalling: Towards the systems level. Nat Rev Mol Cell Biol 2006, Jul;7(7):505-16.

[50] Jänne PA, Engelman JA, Johnson BE. Epidermal growth factor receptor mutations in non-small-cell lung cancer: Implications for treatment and tumor biology. J Clin Oncol 2005, May 10;23(14):3227-34.

[51] Raines EW, Ross R. Platelet-derived growth factor. I. High yield purification and evidence for multiple forms. J Biol Chem 1982, May 10;257(9):5154-60.

[52] Kourembanas S, Morita T, Liu Y, Christou H. Mechanisms by which oxygen regulates gene expression and cell-cell interaction in the vasculature. Kidney Int 1997, Feb;51(2):438-43.

[53] Fredriksson L, Li H, Eriksson U. The PDGF family: Four gene products form five dimeric isoforms. Cytokine Growth Factor Rev 2004, Aug;15(4):197-204.

[54] Roberts WM, Look AT, Roussel MF, Sherr CJ. Tandem linkage of human CSF-1 receptor (c-fms) and PDGF receptor genes. Cell 1988, Nov 18;55(4):655-61.

[55] Heldin CH, Westermark B. Mechanism of action and in vivo role of platelet-derived growth factor. Physiol Rev 1999, Oct;79(4):1283-316.

[56] Zhong H, Chiles K, Feldser D, Laughner E, Hanrahan C, Georgescu MM, et al. Modulation of hypoxia-inducible factor 1alpha expression by the epidermal growth factor/phosphatidylinositol 3-kinase/PTEN/AKT/FRAP pathway in human prostate cancer cells: Implications for tumor angiogenesis and therapeutics. Cancer Res 2000, Mar 15;60(6):1541-5.

[57] Hauck CR, Hsia DA, Schlaepfer DD. Focal adhesion kinase facilitates platelet-derived growth factor-bb-stimulated ERK2 activation required for chemotaxis migration of vascular smooth muscle cells. J Biol Chem 2000, Dec 29;275(52):41092-9.

[58] Keck PJ, Hauser SD, Krivi G, Sanzo K, Warren T, Feder J, Connolly DT. Vascular permeability factor, an endothelial cell mitogen related to PDGF. Science 1989, Dec 8;246(4935):1309-12.

[59] Padhani AR, Krohn KA, Lewis JS, Alber M. Imaging oxygenation of human tumours. Eur Radiol 2007, Apr;17(4):861-72.

[60] Figueiras RG, Padhani AR, Goh VJ, Vilanova JC, González SB, Martín CV, et al. Novel oncologic drugs: What they do and how they affect images. Radiographics 2011;31(7):2059-91.

[61] Provenzale JM. Imaging of angiogenesis: Clinical techniques and novel imaging methods. AJR Am J Roentgenol 2007, Jan;188(1):11-23.

[62] Kambadakone AR, Sahani DV. Body perfusion CT: Technique, clinical applications, and advances. Radiol Clin North Am 2009, Jan;47(1):161-78.

[63] Miles KA, Lee TY, Goh V, Klotz E, Cuenod C, Bisdas S, et al. Current status and guidelines for the assessment of tumour vascular support with dynamic contrast-enhanced computed tomography. European Radiology 2012, Jul;22(7):1430-41.

[64] Ohno Y, Koyama H, Matsumoto K, Onishi Y, Takenaka D, Fujisawa Y, et al. Differentiation of malignant and benign pulmonary nodules with quantitative first-pass 320--detector row perfusion CT versus FDG PET/CT. Radiology 2011;258(2):599-609.

[65] Lind JS, Meijerink MR, Dingemans AM, van Kuijk C, Ollers MC, de Ruysscher D, et al. Dynamic contrast-enhanced CT in patients treated with sorafenib and erlotinib for non-small cell lung cancer: A new method of monitoring treatment? European Radiology 2010, Dec;20(12):2890-8.

[66] Jeswani T, Padhani AR. Imaging tumour angiogenesis. Cancer Imaging 2005;5:131-8.

[67] Ohno Y, Nogami M, Higashino T, Takenaka D, Matsumoto S, Hatabu H, Sugimura K. Prognostic value of dynamic MR imaging for non-small-cell lung cancer patients after chemoradiotherapy. J Magn Reson Imaging 2005, Jun;21(6):775-83.

[68] Johnson DH, Fehrenbacher L, Novotny WF, Herbst RS, Nemunaitis JJ, Jablons DM, et al. Randomized phase II trial comparing bevacizumab plus carboplatin and paclitax-

el with carboplatin and paclitaxel alone in previously untreated locally advanced or metastatic non-small-cell lung cancer. J Clin Oncol 2004, Jun 1;22(11):2184-91.

[69] Sandler A, Gray R, Perry MC, Brahmer J, Schiller JH, Dowlati A, et al. Paclitaxel-carboplatin alone or with bevacizumab for non-small-cell lung cancer. N Engl J Med 2006;355(24):2542-50.

[70] Reck M, von Pawel J, Zatloukal P, Ramlau R, Gorbounova V, Hirsh V, et al. Overall survival with cisplatin-gemcitabine and bevacizumab or placebo as first-line therapy for nonsquamous non-small-cell lung cancer: Results from a randomised phase III trial (avail). Ann Oncol 2010, Sep;21(9):1804-9.

[71] Dansin E, Cinieri S, Garrido P, Griesinger F, Isla D, Koehler M, Kohlhaeufl M. MO19390 (sail): Bleeding events in a phase IV study of first-line bevacizumab with chemotherapy in patients with advanced non-squamous NSCLC. Lung Cancer 2012, Jun;76(3):373-9.

[72] Botrel TEA, Clark O, Clark L, Paladini L, Faleiros E, Pegoretti B. Efficacy of bevacizumab (bev) plus chemotherapy (CT) compared to CT alone in previously untreated locally advanced or metastatic non-small cell lung cancer (NSCLC): Systematic review and meta-analysis. Lung Cancer 2011.

[73] Cao C, Wang J, Bunjhoo H, Xu Y, Fang H. Risk profile of bevacizumab in patients with non-small cell lung cancer: A meta-analysis of randomized controlled trials. Acta Oncol 2012, Feb;51(2):151-6.

[74] Socinski MA, Langer CJ, Huang JE, Kolb MM, Compton P, Wang L, Akerley W. Safety of bevacizumab in patients with non-small-cell lung cancer and brain metastases. J Clin Oncol 2009, Nov 1;27(31):5255-61.

[75] Sandler A, Hirsh V, Reck M, von Pawel J, Akerley W, Johnson DH. An evidence-based review of the incidence of CNS bleeding with anti-vegf therapy in non-small cell lung cancer patients with brain metastases. Lung Cancer 2012, Aug 6.

[76] Kabbinavar FF, Miller VA, et al. Overall survival (OS) in ATLAS, a phase iiib trial comparing bevacizumab (B) therapy with or without erlotinib (E) after completion of chemotherapy (chemo) with B for first-line treatment of locally advanced, recurrent, or metastatic non-small cell lung cancer (NSCLC); J Clin Oncol. ASCO Annual Meeting Proceedings (Post-Meeting Edition): American Society of Clinical Oncology; 2010;28(15s): abstract 7526.

[77] Dahlberg SE, Sandler AB, Brahmer JR, Schiller JH, Johnson DH. Clinical course of advanced non-small-cell lung cancer patients experiencing hypertension during treatment with bevacizumab in combination with carboplatin and paclitaxel on ECOG 4599. J Clin Oncol 2010, Feb 20;28(6):949-54.

[78] Leighl NB, Raez LE, Besse B, Rosen PJ, Barlesi F, Massarelli E, et al. A multicenter, phase 2 study of vascular endothelial growth factor trap (aflibercept) in platinum-

and erlotinib-resistant adenocarcinoma of the lung. J Thorac Oncol 2010, Jul;5(7): 1054-9.

[79] Garon EB, Kabbinavar FF, et al. A randomized phase II trial of a vascular disrupting agent (VDA) fosbretabulin tromethamine (CA4P) with carboplatin (C), paclitaxel (P), and bevacizumab (B) in stage 3B/4 nonsquamous non-small cell lung cancer (NSCLC): Analysis of safety and activity of the FALCON trial; J Clin Oncol. ASCO Annual Meeting Proceedings (Post-Meeting Edition): American Society of Clinical Oncology; 2011;29(15s): abstract 7559.

[80] Mita AC, Heist RS, et al. Phase II study of docetaxel with or without plinabulin (NPI-2358) in patients with non-small cell lung cancer (NSCLC); J Clin Oncol. ASCO Annual Meeting Proceedings (Post-Meeting Edition): American Society of Clinical Oncology; 2010;28(15s): abstract 7592.

[81] McKeage MJ, Von Pawel J, Reck M, Jameson MB, Rosenthal MA, Sullivan R, et al. Randomised phase II study of ASA404 combined with carboplatin and paclitaxel in previously untreated advanced non-small cell lung cancer. Br J Cancer 2008, Dec 16;99(12):2006-12.

[82] Schiller JH, Lee JW, et al. A randomized discontinuation phase II study of sorafenib versus placebo in patients with non-small cell lung cancer who have failed at least two prior chemotherapy regimens: E2501; J Clin Oncol. 2008;26(15s): abstract 8014.

[83] Blumenschein GR, Gatzemeier U, Fossella F, Stewart DJ, Cupit L, Cihon F, et al. Phase II, multicenter, uncontrolled trial of single-agent sorafenib in patients with relapsed or refractory, advanced non-small-cell lung cancer. J Clin Oncol 2009, Sep 10;27(26):4274-80.

[84] Paz-Ares LG, Biesma B, Heigener D, von Pawel J, Eisen T, Bennouna J, et al. Phase III, randomized, double-blind, placebo-controlled trial of gemcitabine/cisplatin alone or with sorafenib for the first-line treatment of advanced, nonsquamous non-small-cell lung cancer. J Clin Oncol 2012, Sep 1;30(25):3084-92.

[85] Scagliotti G, Novello S, von Pawel J, Reck M, Pereira JR, Thomas M, et al. Phase III study of carboplatin and paclitaxel alone or with sorafenib in advanced non-small-cell lung cancer. J Clin Oncol 2010, Apr 10;28(11):1835-42.

[86] Kim ES, Herbst RS, Wistuba II, Lee JJ, Blumenschein GR, Tsao A, et al. The BATTLE trial: Personalizing therapy for lung cancer. Cancer Discov 2011, Jun;1(1):44-53.

[87] Socinski M. Available from: http://clinicaltrials.gov/ct2/show/NCT00693992. Accessed 10 September 2012.

[88] Heymach JV, Paz-Ares L, De Braud F, Sebastian M, Stewart DJ, Eberhardt WE, et al. Randomized phase II study of vandetanib alone or with paclitaxel and carboplatin as first-line treatment for advanced non-small-cell lung cancer. J Clin Oncol 2008, Nov 20;26(33):5407-15.

[89] Heymach JV, Johnson BE, Prager D, Csada E, Roubec J, Pesek M, et al. Randomized, placebo-controlled phase II study of vandetanib plus docetaxel in previously treated non small-cell lung cancer. J Clin Oncol 2007, Sep 20;25(27):4270-7.

[90] Herbst RS, Sun Y, Eberhardt WE, Germonpré P, Saijo N, Zhou C, et al. Vandetanib plus docetaxel versus docetaxel as second-line treatment for patients with advanced non-small-cell lung cancer (ZODIAC): A double-blind, randomised, phase 3 trial. Lancet Oncol 2010, Jul;11(7):619-26.

[91] de Boer RH, Arrieta O, Yang CH, Gottfried M, Chan V, Raats J, et al. Vandetanib plus pemetrexed for the second-line treatment of advanced non-small-cell lung cancer: A randomized, double-blind phase III trial. J Clin Oncol 2011, Mar 10;29(8):1067-74.

[92] Lee JS, Hirsh V, Park K, Qin S, Blajman CR, Perng RP, et al. Vandetanib versus placebo in patients with advanced non-small-cell lung cancer after prior therapy with an epidermal growth factor receptor tyrosine kinase inhibitor: A randomized, double-blind phase III trial (ZEPHYR). J Clin Oncol 2012, Apr 1;30(10):1114-21.

[93] Socinski MA, Novello S, Brahmer JR, Rosell R, Sanchez JM, Belani CP, et al. Multicenter, phase II trial of sunitinib in previously treated, advanced non-small-cell lung cancer. J Clin Oncol 2008, Feb 1;26(4):650-6.

[94] Novello S, Scagliotti GV, Rosell R, Socinski MA, Brahmer J, Atkins J, et al. Phase II study of continuous daily sunitinib dosing in patients with previously treated advanced non-small cell lung cancer. Br J Cancer 2009, Nov 3;101(9):1543-8.

[95] Schiller JH, Larson T, Ou SH, Limentani S, Sandler A, Vokes E, et al. Efficacy and safety of axitinib in patients with advanced non-small-cell lung cancer: Results from a phase II study. J Clin Oncol 2009, Aug 10;27(23):3836-41.

[96] Blumenschein GR, Kabbinavar F, Menon H, Mok TS, Stephenson J, Beck JT, et al. A phase II, multicenter, open-label randomized study of motesanib or bevacizumab in combination with paclitaxel and carboplatin for advanced nonsquamous non-small-cell lung cancer. Ann Oncol 2011, Sep;22(9):2057-67.

[97] Scagliotti GV, Vynnychenko I, Park K, Ichinose Y, Kubota K, Blackhall F, et al. International, randomized, placebo-controlled, double-blind phase III study of motesanib plus carboplatin/paclitaxel in patients with advanced nonsquamous non-small-cell lung cancer: MONET1. J Clin Oncol 2012, Aug 10;30(23):2829-36.

[98] Reck M, Kaiser R, Eschbach C, Stefanic M, Love J, Gatzemeier U, et al. A phase II double-blind study to investigate efficacy and safety of two doses of the triple angiokinase inhibitor BIBF 1120 in patients with relapsed advanced non-small-cell lung cancer. Ann Oncol 2011, Jun;22(6):1374-81.

[99] Wakelee HA, Gettinger SN, Engelman JA. A phase ib/II study of XL184 (BMS 907351) with and without erlotinib (E) in patients (pts) with non-small cell lung cancer (NSCLC); J Clin Oncol. 2010;28(15s): abstract 3017.

Chapter 2

Genetically Engineered Mouse Models for Human Lung Cancer

Kazushi Inoue, Elizabeth Fry, Dejan Maglic and
Sinan Zhu

Additional information is available at the end of the chapter

http://dx.doi.org/10.5772/53721

1. Introduction

Lung cancer is the leading cause of cancer deaths in the world, which is a cause for more solid tumor-related deaths than all other carcinomas combined. More than 170,000 new cases are diagnosed each year in the United States alone, of whom ~160,000 will eventually die, accounting for nearly 30% of all cancer deaths (Siegel *et al.*, 2012). The annual incidence for lung cancer per 100,000 population is highest among African Americans (76.1), followed by whites (69.7), American Indians/Alaska Natives (48.4), and Asian/Pacific Islanders (38.4). Hispanic people have much lower lung cancer incidence (37.3) than non-Hispanics (71.9) (CDC, 2010). These results identify the racial/ethnic populations and geographic regions that would benefit from enhanced efforts in lung cancer prevention, specifically by reducing cigarette smoking and exposure to environmental carcinogens.

Lung lobectomy provides the best chance for patients with early-stage disease to be cured. African American patients with early-stage lung cancer have lower five-year survival rates than whites, which has been attributed to lower rates of resection in former patients (Wisnivesky *et al.*, 2005). Several potential factors underlying racial differences in receiving surgical therapy include differences in pulmonary function, access to care, beliefs about tumor spread at the time of operation, and the possibility of cure without surgery. Of these, access to care is considered to be the most important factor underlying racial disparities.

The most outstanding modifiable risk factor for lung cancer is cigarette smoking (Swierzewski III, 2011). Other risk factors include asbestos exposure, radon, occupational chemicals, radiation, and alcohol. People who smoke tend to drink more alcohols and consume more non-narcotic pain relievers than non-smokers, thus reducing the intoxicating effects of alcohol, promoting the progression from moderate to heavy drinking. Alcoholism is also associated with significant immune suppression - therefore, a history of drinking may increase a person's susceptibility to lung cancer.

Lung cancer has a high morbidity because it is difficult to detect early and is frequently resistant to available chemotherapy and radiotherapy. The overall 5-year survival rate for all types of lung cancer is around 15 % at most, and it is even worse in SCLC (~5 %) although SCLC is more sensitive to chemo/radiation therapy than NSCLC (Meuwissen & Berns, 2005; Schiller, 2001; Worden & Kalemkerian, 2000). Non-smokers who develop lung cancer may experience delays in diagnosis due to the fact that many early symptoms of lung cancer mimic those of non-specific respiratory infections (Menon, 2012). Thus, a physician may misdiagnose the malignant disease for asthma or other respiratory illnesses. Another reason for delayed diagnosis of lung cancer is that there is no sensitive and specific biomarker, such as prostate-specific antigen in prostate cancer (Brambilla *et al.*, 2003). Thus several biomarkers will have to be used together for early diagnosis of lung cancer at present, which include mutant Ras, mutant p53, and methylation of a variety of genes using bronchial biospies or bronchoalveolar lavage (Brambilla *et al.*, 2003).

Certain combinations of clinical signs and symptoms – e.g. endocrine, neurologic, immunologic, and hematologic - are associated with lung cancer as a manifestation of the secretion of cytokines/hormones by tumor cells or as an associated immunologic response (Yeung *et al.*, 2011). These paraneoplastic syndromes occur commonly in patients with SCLC. Since the syndromes can be the first clinical manifestation of malignant disease, increased awareness of these syndromes associated with lung cancer is critical to the earlier diagnosis of malignancies, thereby improving the overall prognosis of patients.

Lung cancer has been categorized into two major histopathological groups: non-small-cell lung cancer (NSCLC) (Moran, 2006) and small-cell lung cancer (SCLC) (Schiller, 2001), the latter of which show neuroendocrine features and thus are different from the former. Approximately 80 % of lung cancers are NSCLC, and they are subcategorized into adenocarcinomas (AdCA), squamous cell (SqCLC), bronchioalveolar, and large-cell carcinomas (LCLC) (Travis, 2002). SCLC and NSCLC show major differences in histopathologic characteristics that can be explained by the distinct patterns of genetic alterations found in both tumor types (Zochbauer-Muller *et al*., 2002). The *K-Ras* gene is mutated in 20~30 % of NSCLC while its mutation is rare in SCLC; *Rb* inactivation is found in ~90 % of SCLC while $p16^{INK4a}$ is inactivated by gene deletion and/or promoter hypermethylation in ~50 % of NSCLC (Fong *et al.*, 2003; Meuwissen & Berns, 2005). Responsiveness of tumor cells to chemotherapy and/or radiation therapy significantly varies between NSCLC and SCLC, and thus, has a dramatic effect on the prognosis of patients.

Progress in whole genome approaches to detect genetic alterations found in human lung cancer has resulted in the identification of a growing number of genes. Genome-wide association studies, whether they are based on single-nucleotide polymorphism array or in gene copy number assays, have identified mutations in lung cancer-related genes. Identification of these lung cancer-related genes will provide great potential as therapeutic targets for lung cancer intervention. Target validation should be done through intervention studies of specific genetic alterations in human lung cancer cell lines. Since *in vitro* cell culture studies cannot fully mimic more complex *in vivo* onset/development of lung carcinogenesis, developing endogenous lung cancer in mice that harbor specific mutations will undoubtedly provide a further insight into the mutation-specific effects on lung tumor initiation/development. Moreover, a high degree of pathophysiological similarity between mouse lung tumors and human lung carcinomas will make it possible to use these mouse models in pre-clinical tests for novel anticancer drug screening. Various intervention strategies against specific mutation can then be tested to evaluate both specificity and efficacy in mouse lung tumors at every developing stage. The number of genetically engineered mouse models for lung cancer is ever expanding. Continuous attempt to manipulate the mouse genome has enabled us to adjust compound mouse models of lung cancer in a way that they start to reproduce the more complex human lung cancer in a higher degree.

While susceptibility and incidence of spontaneous lung tumors vary among well-established mouse strains, endogenous mouse lung tumors share many similarities with human lung cancers. This was clearly demonstrated in early studies where defined chemical carcinogens were used to induce lung tumors in mice (Wakamatsu *et al.*, 2007). The incidence of spontaneous and induced lung tumors were very high (61%) in A/J and SWR strains, but very low (6%) in resistant strains such as C57BL/6 and DBA (Wakamatsu *et al.*, 2007). Contrary to human lung cancer with its complex molecular genetics and four distinct tumor types (adenocarcinoma, squamous cell carcinoma, large-cell carcinoma, and small-cell carcinoma) that easily metastasize, spontaneous and chemically-induced lung lesions in mice often result in pulmonary adenomas and more infrequent adenocarcinomas. Mouse lung adenocarcinomas are usually 5mm or more in diameter; however, they are categorized into carcinomas when nuclear atypia or signs of local invasion/metastasis is found in tumors less than 5mm. Mouse lung tumor development shows initial hyperplastic foci in bronchioles and alveoli, which then become benign adenomas and eventually adenocarcinomas (Shimkin *et al.*, 1975). The tumor latency depends on mouse strain and carcinogen administration protocols. Most potent carcinogens are found in cigarettes, such as polycyclic aromatic hydrocarbons, tobacco-specific nitrosamine, and benzopyrene (BaP) (Pfeifer *et al.*, 2002). It has been especially difficult to reproduce well-characterized pre-malignant lesions found in human airway epithelium in mice (Sato *et al.*, 2007). Nevertheless, major histopathological features remain the same between the two species and molecular characterization of spontaneous and carcinogen-induced murine lung tumors revealed a high degree of similarity as compared to their human counterparts (Malkinson, 2001). A common early event is the occurrence of activating *K-ras* mutations in hyperplastic lesions. Besides overexpression of c-*Myc*, inactivation of well-known tumor suppressor genes, such as *p53*, *fhit*, *Apc*, *Rb*, *Mcc*, $p16^{Ink4a}$ and/or *Arf* occur in both mice and human lung cancers; only a small percentage of lung adenomas progress into AdCAs (Malkinson, 2001).

2. The first generation mouse models for lung cancer

The first generation transgenic models for lung cancer were created by ectopic transgene expression under control of lung-specific promoters. Thus transgenic expression was constitutive. Transgene expression was mainly found in specific subsets of lung epithelial cells. Lung *surfactant protein C* (*SPC*) promoter was used for constitutive gene expression in type II alveolar cells whereas *Clara Cell Secretory Protein* (*CCSP*) promoter was used to target the non-ciliated secretory (Clara) cells that exist on the airways. In early studies, *SV40 Tag* (Simian virus large T-antigen) that neutralizes the activity of both Rb and p53 was constitutively expressed under the control of *CCSP* (DeMayo *et al.*, 1991; Sandmoller *et al.*, 1994) or *SPC* promoters (Wikenheiser *et al.*, 1992). Although each tumor originated from either Clara cells or type II alveolar cells, they both resulted in quite similar aggressive AdCAs without metastases (Wikenheiser *et al.*, 1997). A similar strategy was used to express distinct oncogenes (such as *c-Raf* and *c-Myc* [Geick *et al.*, 2001]) in the lung/bronchial epithelium, ending up with a milder phenotype, as both transgenic mice mainly developed adenomas, and a few progressed to AdCAs without any metastases.

Ehrhardt *et al.* (2001) created transgenic mouse models to study tumorigenesis of bronchiolo-alveolar AdCAs derived from alveolar type II pneumocytes. Transgenic lines expressing c-*Myc* under the control of the *SPC* promoter developed multifocal bronchiolo-alveolar hyperplasias, adenomas, AdCAs, whereas transgenic lines expressing a secretable form of the epidermal growth factor, TGFα, developed hyperplasias of the alveolar epithelium. Since the oncogenes c-Myc and TGFα are frequently overexpressed in human lung bronchiolo-alveolar carcinomas, these mouse lines will be useful as those for human lung bronchiolo-alveolar carcinomas (Ehrhardt *et al.*, 2001).

Sunday *et al.* created a transgenic model for primary pulmonary neuroendocrine cell hyperplasia/neoplasia using *v-Ha-ras* driven by the *neuroendocrine* (NE)-specific calcitonin promoter (named *rascal*). All rascal transgenic mouse lineages developed hyperplasias of NE and non-NE cells, but mostly non-NE cells developed lung carcinomas (Sunday *et al.*, 1999). Analyses of embryonic lung demonstrated *rascal* mRNA in undifferentiated epithelium, consistent with expression in a common pluripotent precursor cell. These observations indicate that *v-Ha-ras* can lead to both NE and non-NE hyperplasia/carcinoma *in vivo* (Sunday *et al.*, 1999).

A strong correlation exists between *p53* mutations and lung malignancies, and LOH for *p53* has been reported in 40% of NSCLC with specific primers (Mallakin *et* al., 2007). Preceding this study, Morris *et al.* (1998) established a transgenic mouse model with disrupted p53 function in the epithelial cells of the peripheral lung. A dominant-negative mutant form of *p53* was expressed from the human *SPC* promoter. The dominant-negative p53 (dnp53) expressed from the *SPC* promoter antagonized wild-type p53 functions in alveolar type II pneumocytes and some bronchiolar cells of the transgenic animals, and thereby promoted the development of carcinoma of the lung. This mouse model should prove useful to the study of lung carcinogenesis and to the identification of agents that contribute to neoplastic conversion in the lung. Another group later created *CCSP-dnp53* transgenic mice and reported significant increase in the incidence of spontaneous lung cancer in 18-month-old transgenic mice (Tchon-Wong *et al.*, 2002). In addition to the increased incidence of spontaneous lung tumor, these transgenic mice were more susceptible to the development of lung adenocarcinoma after exposure to BaP. The risk of lung tumors was 25.3 times greater in BaP-treated mice adjusted for transgene expression. These results suggest that p53 function is important for protecting mice from both spontaneous and BaP-induced lung cancers.

http://dx.doi.org/10.5772/53721

The receptor tyrosine kinase RON (recepteur d'origine nantais) is a member of the MET proto-oncogene family, which is expressed by a variety of epithelial-derived tumors and cancer cell lines and has been implicated in the pathogenesis of lung adenocarcinomas (Chen *et al.*, 2002). To determine the oncogenic potential of RON, transgenic mice were generated using the lung *SPC* promoter to express human wild-type RON in type II cell phenotypes (Chen *et al.*, 2002). The mice were born normal without morphological alterations in the lung, however, multiple adenomas appeared as a single mass in the lung around 2 months of age and gradually developed into multiple nodules throughout the lung. Most of the tumors were characterized as cuboidal epithelial cells with type II cell phenotypes which transformed from pre-malignant adenomas to adenocarcinomas. Interestingly, Ras expression was dramatically increased in the majority of tumors without mutation in the 'hot spots' of the *K-Ras* or *p53* genes suggesting that *SPC-RON* is a mouse lung tumor model with unique biological characteristics (Chen *et al.*, 2002).

Many prominent genetic lesions found in human lung cancer clearly link the inactivation of well-known tumor suppressor genes (Sekido *et al.*, 2003) to lung cancer development. Initial attempts to mimic some of these lesions implicated in lung cancer by using conventional knockout mice had limited success with respect to the onset of lung cancer. The main reason for this failure was that germ-line deletion of many essential tumor suppressor genes (such as the *retinoblastoma* gene (*Rb*) (Jacks *et al.*, 1992) lead to embryonal lethality. Non-essential tumor suppressor gene (for embryonic survival) knockout mice often had a very broad tumor spectrum of which lung tumors formed only a minor fraction. Thus, *p53*, $p16^{Ink4a}$ and $p19^{Arf}$ (Meuwissen & Berns, 2005) null allele mice seldom develop lung AdCAs. However, introducing similar mutations into endogenous *p53* alleles, such as those prominently found in Li–Fraumeni patients, generated $p53^{R270H/+}$ and $p53^{R172H/+}$ which had a different tumor spectrum compared with $p53^{+/-}$ mice (Olive *et al.*, 2004), although their mean survival times were identical. Interestingly these mice, but especially $p53^{R270H/+}$ and $p53^{R270H/-}$ mice, gave rise to more malignant lung AdCAs, and even their metastases, which never occurred in $p53^{-/-}$ mice. These results suggest that "humanized" *p53* mutations have a greater impact on lung tumor progression than complete *p53* loss (Olive *et al.*, 2004; Lang *et al.*, 2004).

Targeting genes deleted early in human lung tumorigenesis, such as the complete cluster at chromosome 3p21.3, showed that heterozygous deletion for this 370 kb region showed no obvious predisposition for lung cancer development albeit homozygous deletion caused embryonal lethality (Smith *et al.*, 2002). A more specific deletion of candidate tumor suppressor genes on chromosome 3 like *RassF1a*, *FHIT* and *VHL*, showed that 31% of $Rassf1a^{-/-}$ mice produced spontaneous mainly lymphomas but also lung adenomas (Tommasi *et al.*, 2005). Treatment of $Rassf1a^{-/-}$ mice with BP or urethane resulted in an even higher rate of lung tumors. No spontaneous lung tumors were observed in $Fhit^{-/-}$ or $Vhl^{+/-}$ mice, but 44% of $Fhit^{-/-};Vhl^{+/-}$ mice developed AdCAs by age 2 years. Again use of mutagens such as dimethylnitrosamine led to 100% adenoma and AdCA induction in $Fhit^{-/-};Vhl^{+/-}$ mice and even adenomas in 40% of $Fhit^{-/-}$ mice by age 20 months (Zanesi *et al.*, 2005). This showed the usefulness of these knockout mice in recapitulating a pattern of early lung cancer development similar to human pattern.

3. The second generation models

3.1. K-ras^{LA} and LSL K-ras models

A different approach to address lung cancer onset was the use of knock-in alleles to activate oncogenes. One example of this is based on the somatic *K-ras* activation *via* an oncogenic *Kras^{G12D}* knock-in allele (*Kras^{LA2}*), which is expressed only after a spontaneous recombination event (Johnson *et al.*, 2001). In this way, sporadic Kras^{G12D} expression occurred on an endogenous level, which in turn augments efficient development of lung AdCAs. However, these mice also developed other tumor lesions as K-Ras^{G12D} expression was not limited to the lung epithelial tissues.

Dmp1 (Dmtf1) is a Myb-like protein with tumor suppressive activity that had been isolated in a yeast two-hybrid screen with cyclin D2 bait (Hirai and Sherr, 1996; Inoue and Sherr, 1998; for review, Inoue *et al.*, 2007; Sugiyama *et al.*, 2008a). The promoter is activated by oncogenic Ras-Raf signaling and induces cell-cycle arrest in an Arf, p53-dependent fashion (Inoue *et al.*, 1999; Sreeramaneni *et al.*, 2005). Both *Dmp1$^{+/-}$* and *Dmp1$^{-/-}$* mice are prone to spontaneous and carcinogen-induced tumor development, indicating that it is haplo-insufficient for tumor suppression, the mechanism of which have not been elucidated yet (Inoue *et al.*, 2000, 2001, 2007). The survival of *K-ras^{LA}* mice was shortened by approximately 15 weeks in both *Dmp1$^{+/-}$* and *Dmp1$^{-/-}$* backgrounds, the lung tumors of which showed significantly decreased frequency of *p53* mutations compared to *Dmp1$^{+/+}$*. Approximately 40% of *K-ras^{LA}* lung tumors from *Dmp1* wild-type mice lost one allele of the *Dmp1* gene, suggesting the primary involvement of *Dmp1* in *K-ras*-induced tumorigenesis (Mallakin *et al.*, 2007). Tumors from *Dmp1*-deficient mice showed more invasive and aggressive phenotypes than those from *Dmp1* wild-type mice. Loss of heterozygosity (LOH) of the h*DMP1* locus was detectable in approximately 35% of human lung carcinomas, which was found in mutually exclusive fashion with LOH of *INK4a/ARF* or that of *p53*. Thus, *DMP1* is a novel tumor suppressor for both human and murine NSCLC (Mallakin *et al.*, 2007; Sugiyama *et al.*, 2008b).

Integration of gene expression data from a *Kras^{LA2}* mouse model and *KRAS* mutated human lung tumors showed a significant overlap but also revealed a gene-expression signature for *K-ras* mutation in human lung cancer itself (Sweet-Cordero *et al.*, 2005). By using *Kras^{LA2}* knock-in mouse model and human lung cancer specimen, they compared gene expression patterns between these two species (Sweet-Cordero *et al.*, 2005). They applied this method to the analysis of a model of *Kras^{LA2}*-mediated lung cancer and found a good relationship to human lung AdCA, thereby validating the usefulness of this transgenic model. Furthermore, integrating mouse and human data uncovered a gene-expression signature of *KRAS2* mutation in human lung cancer. They confirmed the importance of this signature by gene-expression analysis of shRNA-mediated inhibition of oncogenic *Kras^{LA2}* (Sweet-Cordero *et al.*, 2005). However, one problem of *Kras^{LA}* mice is that they develop tumors other than lung cancer (Mallakin *et al.*, 2007). To overcome this issue, Jackson *et al.* (2001) developed a new model of lung AdCA in mice having a conditionally activatable allele of oncogenic *K-ras* (*LSL Kras^{G12D}*). They show that the use of a recombinant adenovirus expressing Cre recombinase (AdenoCre) to induce *Kras^{G12D}* expression in the lungs of mice allows control of the tim-

http://dx.doi.org/10.5772/53721

ing and multiplicity of tumor initiation. Through the ability to synchronize tumor initiation in these mice, they could characterize the stages of tumor progression. Of particular significance, this system led to the identification of a new cell type contributing to the development of pulmonary AdCA (Jackson *et al.*, 2001). By using this Cre-lox system, the same group later created conditional knock-in mice with mutations in *K-ras* combined with one of mutant *p53* alleles (Jackson *et al.*, 2005). *p53*-loss strongly promoted the progression of *Kras*-induced lung AdCAs, yielding a mouse model that precisely recapitulates advanced human lung AdCA. The influence of *p53*-loss on malignant progression was observed as early as 6 weeks after tumor initiation. They also found that the contact mutant p53R270H behaved in a dominant-negative fashion to promote *K-ras*-driven lung AdCAs. Of note, a subset of mice also developed sinonasal adenocarcinomas, suggesting specific expression of *K-ras* in this tissue. In contrast to the lung tumors, expression of the point-mutant *p53* alleles strongly promoted the development of sinonasal AdCAs compared with simple loss-of-function, suggesting a tissue-specific gain-of-function of mutant p53 (Jackson *et al.*, 2005).

Since activating *K-ras* mutation models recapitulate the human lung tumor phenotypes well, closer analyses of early lung tumor initiating events were performed (Ji *et al.*, 2006). A combination of both *CCSP-Cre* recombinase and *LSL* $Kras^{G12D}$ alleles (Jackson *et al.*, 2005) resulted in a progressive phenotype of cellular atypia, adenoma and finally AdCA. The activation of *K-ras* mutant allele in CC10-positive cells resulted in a progressive phenotype characterized by cellular atypia, adenoma and ultimately AdCA. Surprisingly, *Kras* activation in the bronchiolar epithelium was associated with a robust inflammatory response characterized by an abundant infiltration of alveolar macrophages and neutrophils. These mice displayed early mortality in the setting of this pulmonary inflammatory response. Bronchoalveolar lavage fluid from these mutant mice contained the MIP-2, KC, MCP-1 and LIX chemokines that increased significantly with age. Thus, *Kras* activation in the lung induces inflammatory chemokines and provides an excellent means to study the complex interactions between inflammatory cells, chemokines, and tumor progression (Ji *et al.*, 2006).

3.2. Doxycycline (dox)-inducible/de-inducible lung cancer models

In $Kras^{LA}$ mice, oncogene can be induced, but it cannot be de-induced after lung carcinogenesis. To improve this mouse model, a better method of replicating gene expression patterns of target oncogenes had to be taken into account. Furthermore, a general knock-in or knockout procedure only poorly represents genetic events that occur during sporadic lung cancer since genes are already deleted already *in utero* (Jonkers & Berns, 2002). Conditional regulation of the temporal-spatial expression of oncogenes or inactivation of tumor suppressor genes in somatic tissues of choice can more accurately mimic the *in vivo* situation leading to the onset of sporadic cancer (Jonkers & Berns, 2002; Lewandoski, 2001). This is why the second generation of mouse models for lung cancer makes use of a conditional bitransgenic tet-inducible system (Lewandoski, 2001). Most often, the reverse tetracycline (tet)-controlled transactivator (*rt*TA) inducible system is used. The first transgene with the *rt*TA element behind a tissue-specific promoter causes the *rt*TA expression in a specific cell types, e.g. MMTV-*rt*TA, CCSP-*rt*TA. This transgene is then combined with a second transgene, consisting of a target gene behind a tet-responsive promoter (*tetO*$_7$) vector, e.g. pTRE-Tight (2nd generation vector from Clontech). The presence of tet/dox ensures stable interaction of the *rt*TA element with the *tetO*$_7$ promoter, which, in turn, expresses the target gene upon exposure to tet or dox.

Therefore, on/off target gene expression is possible depending on administration or withdrawal of tet/dox (Gossen *et al.*, 1992). Both *SPC-rtTA* and *CCSP-rtTA* transgenes (Perl *et al.*, 2002) have been used for directing dox-responsive *rt*TA to either alveolar type II or Clara cells. Although both of these promoters have been used to create lung cancer models of mice, CCSP-*rt*TA has more widely been used than SPC-*rt*TA since the *CCSP* promoter is active in both Clara cells and alveolar type II cells while the *SPC* promoter is active only in alveolar type II cells (Floyd *et al.*, 2005). Several transgenic mice such as *CCSP-rtTA;tetO*$_7$*-FGF-7* and *CCSP-rtTA;tetO*$_7$*-Kras*^{G12D} have been successfully created to induce lung lesions in response to antibiotics (Tichelaar *et al.*, 2000; Fisher *et al.*, 2001). Induction of FGF-7 caused initial epithelial cell hyperplasia followed by adenomatous hyperplasia after dox application. All hyperplasia disappeared after withdrawal of dox (Tichelaar *et al.*, 2000). However, mouse Kras^{G12D} induction caused epithelial cell hyperplasia, adenomatous hyperplasia and, after 2 months dox application, multiple adenomas and AdCAs. Again, no lesion was detected after 1 month of dox withdrawal (Fisher *et al.*, 2001). When the *CCSP-rtTA;tetO*$_7$ *Kras*^{G12D} alleles were combined with conventional *p53* or *Ink4a/Arf*-null alleles, AdCAs with a more malignant phenotype appeared after 1 month dox treatment, thus showing a synergy of mutant *K-ras* and *p53* or *Ink4a/Arf* deficiencies. However, even in these compound *tet*-inducible mouse models, all lesions disappeared after dox withdrawal. This finding demonstrated the importance of mutant *K-ras* as a "driving" oncogene not only at tumor onset, but also during maintenance of AdCA in these mice (Fisher *et al.*, 2001).

Other models for early, benign lung tumor lesions have been created by using a bitransgenic *tet*-inducible human *Kras*^{G12C} allele that can be expressed in both Clara and/or alveolar type II cells (Tichelaar *et al.*, 2000; Floyd *et al.*, 2005). Expression of human Kras^{G12C} caused multiple, small lung tumors over a 12-month time period. Although tumor multiplicity increased upon continued *K-ras* expression, most lung lesions were hyperplasias or well-differentiated adenomas (Floyd *et al.*, 2005). This is in good contrast to the more severe phenotypes observed in other transgenic mouse models in which different mutant *K-ras* alleles were expressed in the lung. Expression of K-ras^{G12C} was associated with a 2-fold increase in the activation of the Ras and Ral signaling pathways and increased phosphorylation of Ras downstream effectors, including Erk, p90 ribosomal S6 kinase, ribosomal S6 protein, p38 and MAPKAPK-2. In contrast, expression of K-ras^{G12C} had no effect on the activation of the JNK and Akt signaling pathways explaining low tumor induction by human *Kras*^{G12C}. This observation was in strong contrast to the effects of the previously described mouse *Kras*^{G12D} models (Fisher et al., 2001).

3.3. Cre/loxP or Flp/Frt models

The *Cre/loxP* or *Flp/FRT* system (Jonkers & Berns, 2002; Lewandoski, 2001; Dutt *et al.*, 2006) provided excellent tools for reproducing more complicated lung tumor genetics found in

http://dx.doi.org/10.5772/53721

human lung cancers, by introducing somatic mutations in a limited number of differentiated cells of choice whereby other cells of the fully developed lung remained normal. In short, mutations of targeted regions, flanked by loxP (also known as being "floxed") or flippase recombination target (Frt) sequence sites, were introduced through deletion by their respective site-specific recombinases Cre or Flp. Thus, in the case of tumor suppressor genes, conditional hypomorphic mutations (i.e., lower than normal function of the protein) or null allele, several coding or non-coding exons are floxed and can, therefore, be deleted by its corresponding recombinase. Conversely, floxed transcription stops (Lox-Stop-Lox or LSL) in front of oncogene or knock-in alleles can control their respective conditional activation (Jackson *et al.*, 2001) as in the case of *LSL* $KRas^{G12D}$ mice described in the previous section.

The determining factor of this conditional approach is the control of temporal-spatial Cre or FRT recombinase expression. For that purpose, several *Cre* transgenic lines have been generated, with or without *tet*-inducible promoters (Perl *et al.*, 2002). Apart from this, Cre-mediated recombination can also be achieved through the administration of an engineered Adeno-Cre virus *via* nasal or tracheal inhalation (Meuwissen *et al.*, 2001; Jackson *et al.*, 2001). An advantage of the latter method is that a limited amount of adult lung cells can be targeted in a very concise, localized, and timely fashion. Efficacy of this method was tested with conditional alleles of $KRas^{G12D}$ and $KRas^{G12V}$ (Jackson *et al.*, 2001; Guerra *et al.*, 2003). Infection of adult lungs with Adeno-Cre virus rapidly resulted in the onset of adenomatous alveolar hyperplasia, followed by the development of adenomas and AdCAs at 3-4 months post-infection. Although a latency of 8 months was also observed (Guerra *et al.*, 2003), no metastases could be found in any of the models. Most probably a single *K-ras* activation is not enough to allow the AdCAs to progress into a higher state of malignancy as would be required for fully metastasizing lesions. However, these straightforward experiments disclosed the important role of *K-ras* in human lung cancer onset and progression (Guerra *et al.*, 2003). Another important aspect of this model was that lung tumor multiplicity could be controlled by the dose of *Adeno-Cre* virus infecting only a subset of lung epithelial cells. This, together with a controlled time-point of *Adeno-Cre* application, mimics sporadic character of human lung cancer development. However, one has to be careful to note that variability of the *Adeno-Cre* virus delivery and infection (especially with the intranasal method) might lead to inconsistent experimental results. Nevertheless this versatile method remains powerful in that it resembles human lung cancer events.

4. Specific oncogenes in mouse lung cancer models

4.1. Kras downstream effectors and lung cancer – Roles of Raf

Since *Kras* mutations are very common (20-25%) in NSCLC, the understanding of the precise signaling cascade of the Kras pathway is very important (Ji *et al.*, 2007). One of the best characterized Ras pathways is Ras/Raf/MEK/ERK. In fact, *BRAF* gene mutations have been found in a variety of human cancers including NSCLC (Davies *et al.*, 2002; Ji *et al.*, 2007). Oncogenic mutations of *BRAF* render constitutively phosphorylation of the protein, resulting in continued ERK activation. Of all the *BRAF* mutations, *BRAF-V600E* is the most frequent. (Mercer *et al.*, 2003). Dankort *et al.* (2007) created BRaf(CA) (CA: constitutively active) mice to express normal BRaf prior to Cre-mediated recombination after which *BRaf(V600E)* was expressed at physiological levels. *BRaf(CA)* mice infected with an Adenovirus expressing Cre recombinase developed benign lung tumors that only rarely progressed to AdCA. The reason for this is the initial proliferation is halted by increased expression of senescence markers p53 and Ink4a/Arf. Consistent with the tumor suppressor function for Ink4a/Arf and p53, BRaf(V600E) expression combined with mutation of either locus led to lung cancer progression. Moreover, *BRaf(VE)*-induced lung tumors were prevented by pharmacological inhibition of MEK1/2.

In another study, Ji *et al* generated a lung-specific, *tet*-inducible, mice model in which the *CCSP-rtTA;tetO₇-BRAFV600E* induced a development of lung AdCA with bronchioalveolar carcinoma type. The extracellular signal-regulated kinase (ERK)-1/2 (MAPK) pathway was highly activated by the expression of *BRAF(V600E)* mutant. Upon dox withdrawal, the deinduction of *BRAF*-mutant expression led to regression of lung tumors together with a marked decrease in phosphorylation of ERK1/2. Furthermore, the *in vivo* use of a specific MAPK/ERK kinase (MEK) inhibitor also induced lung tumor regression. All these results showed that both activated BRAF and KRAS signaling converge onto the same MAPK pathway, making this pathway a potential target for lung tumor intervention.

The significance of c-Raf was also investigated in *K-Ras*^{G12V}-driven NSCLCs. Ablation of c-Raf in *K-Ras*$^{+/G12V}$; *c-Raf*$^{lox/lox}$ mice induced dramatic increase of survival rate and life span due to the decrease of tumor burden. This result suggests the essential role of c-Raf in mediating oncogenic Ras signaling in NSCLCs (Blasco *et al*, 2011).

Further investigation during *Kras*^{G12D}-driven lung tumorigenesis showed the MAPK antagonist Sprouty-2 (Spry-2) was upregulated. When *Spry-2* was knocked out in Cre/lox dependent *Spry-2*$^{flox/flox}$;*LSL Kras*^{G12D} mice, both tumor number and total tumor area were significantly increased. This clearly suggested a tumor suppressor activity for *Sprouty-2* during *Kras*-dependent lung tumorigenesis by involving in antagonism of Ras/MAPK signaling (Shaw *et al.*, 2007).

By using *CCSP-rtTA;TetO-Cre;LSL-Kras(G12D)*mice Cho *et al.* (2011) established a dox-inducible, Kras(G12D)-driven lung AdCA to pursue the cellular origin and molecular processes involved in *Kras*-induced tumorigenesis. The EpCAM(+)MHCII(-) cells (bronchiolar origin) were more enriched with tumorigenic cells in generating secondary tumors than EpCAM(+)MHCII(+) cells (alveolar origin). In addition, secondary tumors derived from EpCAM(+)MHCII(-) cells showed diversity of tumor locations compared with those derived from EpCAM(+)MHCII(+) cells. Secondary tumors from EpCAM(+)MHCII(-) cells expressed differentiation marker, pro-SPC, consistent with the notion that cancer-initiating cells display not only the abilities for self-renewal, but also the features of differentiation to generate tumors of heterogeneous phenotypes. High level of ERK1/2 activation and colony-forming ability as well as lack of Sprouty-2 expression were also observed in EpCAM(+)MHCII(-) cells. Their data suggested that bronchiolar Clara cells are the origin of tumorigenic cells for Kras(G12D)-induced lung cancer.

4.2. PI3K and lung cancer

Another important pro-survival pathway that is interlinked with RAS is PI3K/Akt signaling pathway. Phosphoinositide-3-kinase (PI3K) consists of a regulatory (p85) and a catalytic (p110) subunit. The overexpression of both subunits was reported in lung carcinomas (Samuels & Velculescu 2004; Wojtalla *et al.*, 2011). Furthermore, selective *PIK3CA* amplification was found in lung squamous cell carcinomas (Angulo *et al.*, 2008). To investigate the oncogenic potential of PIK3CA, transgenic mice were generated with a *tet*-inducible expression of an activated p110α mutant, H1047R, and it was crossed with CCSP-*rt*TA mice to generate *CCSP-rtTA;tetO*$_7$*;PIK3CA(H1047R)* compound mice. Upon dox treatment of animals for 14 weeks, double transgenic mice developed AdCAs, which subsequently disappeared after dox withdrawal for 3 weeks (Engelman *et al.*, 2008). To identify the effect of loss of PI3K signaling in *Kras*-induced lung tumorigenesis, PI3K activity was completely eliminated in *p85* knockouts (*Pik3r2*$^{-/-}$*;Pik3r1*$^{-/-}$), and a dramatic decrease in the number of lung tumors was observed in *LSL Kras*^{G12D}*;Pik3r2*$^{-/-}$*;Pik3r1*$^{-/-}$ mice (Engelman *et al.*, 2008). The clinical efficacy of NVP-BEZ235, a dual pan-PI3K and mammalian target of rapamycin (mTOR) inhibitor was also evaluated against p110α H1047R-induced mouse lung tumors. Application of this drug led to marked tumor regression. In contrast, NVP-BEZ235 barely had effect on mouse lung cancers driven by mutant *Kras*. However, a combination of NVP-BEZ235 and a MEK inhibitor ARRY-142886, had marked synergistic effect on tumor regression. These *in vivo* studies suggest that inhibitors of the PI3K-mTOR pathway when combined with MEK inhibitors, may effectively treat KRAS mutated lung cancers. Of note, Ras proteins directly interact with the p110α subunit of PI3K and introduction of specific mutations (T208D and K227A) in *PIK3CA* blocks this interaction (Gupta *et al.*, 2007). To study the Ras-p110α interactions *in vivo* and its effects on tumorigenesis, these point mutations were introduced into the *Pik3ca* gene in the mice and these mice were crossed with *Kras*^{LA2} alleles (Gupta *et al.*, 2007). Interestingly, they were highly resistant to *Kras* induced lung tumor development, which suggest Ras-p110α interaction is required for Ras-driven tumorigenesis (Gupta *et al.*, 2007). All these results emphasize the importance of PI3K signaling, not only in lung tumor induction, but also maintenance.

4.3. Rac and lung cancer

Rac is a member of the Rho family of small GTPases, and it mediates the regulation of various important cellular processes including cell migration, proliferation and adhesion, all of which may contribute to tumorigenesis (Mack *et al.*, 2011). The important role of Rac in Ras induced lung tumorigenesis was demonstrated in a mice model in which an oncogenic allele of *Kras* was activated by Cre-mediated recombination in the presence or absence of conditional deletion of *Rac1*. They showed that Rac1 function was required for tumorigenesis in lung carcinogenesis for mice with *Rac1* deletion had tumor regression and longer survival. These data showed a specific requirement for Rac1 function in cells expressing oncogenic *K-ras* (Kissil *et al.*, 2007).

4.4. Receptor-type protein tyrosine kinase and lung cancer – Roles of EGFR

4.4.1. EGFR and lung cancer

Epidermal growth factor (EGF) receptor family is one type of RTKs, on which the tyrosine residues phosphorylation lead to activation of downstream TK signaling that contributes to cell proliferation, motility and invasion (Stella *et al.*, 2012). The activation mutations on *EGFR* gene are found in about 10-20% of advanced NSCLC cases and its protein overexpression is found in more than 60% of all lung cancers (Lynch *et al.*, 2004; Soria, *et al.*, 2012). Lynch *et al.* reported that EGFR mutation correlated with clinical responsiveness to the tyrosine kinase inhibitor gefitinib (2004). Since these mutations lead to increased growth factor signaling with susceptibility to the inhibitor, screening for such mutations in lung cancers will identify patients who will have a response to gefitinib. To study a specific oncogenic potential of *EGFR* mutant, the variant III (vIII) deletion, Ji *et al.* (2006a) produced *Tet-op-EGFRvIII; CCSP-rtTA* mice, in which the EGFRvIII expression was induced in lung type II pneumocytes upon dox administration. Mice developed atypical adenomatous hyperplasia after 6-8 weeks of dox induction and progressed to lung adenocarcinomas after 16 weeks with high activation of AKT and ERK signaling pathways. De-induction of EGFRvIII resulted in significant tumor regression, supporting the requirement of continuous EGFRvIII expression in lung tumorigenesis. Furthermore, by using an EGFR/ERB2 inhibitor HKI-272, they found tumor volume in *EGFRvIII ; CCSP-rtTA; Ink4a/Arf*$^{-/-}$ mice was dramatically decreased, suggesting a therapeutic strategy for lung cancers with *EGFRvIII* mutation by an irreversible EGFR inhibitor (Ji *et al.*, 2006a). Politi *et al.* (2006) also studied the role of EGFR mutations in the initiation and maintenance of lung cancer, and developed transgenic mice that express an exon 19 deletion mutant (EGFR(ΔL747-S752)) or the L858R mutant (EGFR(L858R)) in type II pneumocytes under the control of dox, and reported that expression of either EGFR mutant lead to the development of lung AdCa. Ji *et al.* (2006b) later created bitransgenic mice with inducible expression in type II pneumocytes of two common hEGFR mutants (hEGFR^{DEL} and hEGFR^{L858R}) seen in human lung cancer. Both bitransgenic lines developed lung AdCa with hEGFR mutant expression, confirming their oncogenic potential. Maintenance of transformed phenotypes of these lung cancers was dependent on sustained expression of the EGFR mutants. Treatment with small molecule inhibitors (erlotinib or HKI-272) as well as a humanized anti-hEGFR antibody (cetuximab) led to dramatic tumor regression (Ji *et al.*, 2006b). Thus persistent EGFR signaling is required for tumor maintenance in human lung AdCas expressing EGFR mutants. Li *et al.* (2007) generated another dox-inducible lung cancer mice model harboring both erlotinib sensitizing and resistence mutations L858R and T790M (*EGFR TL*). They found that specific expression of *EGFR TL* in lung compartments led to the development of typical bronchioloalveolar carcinoma after 4-5 weeks and peripheral adenocarcinoma after 7-9 weeks. Treatment of *EGFR TL*-driven tumors is most effective when using combined regimen of HKI-272 and rapamycin, suggesting that this combination therapy may benefit pateints harboring erlotinib resistence EGFR mutation (Li *et al.*, 2007).

http://dx.doi.org/10.5772/53721

4.5. HER2 and lung cancer

The c-*ERBB2* gene is located on chromosome 17q11.2-12 and encodes **H**uman **E**pidermal Growth Factor **R**eceptor **2** (HER2) (Hu *et al.*, 2011). This is a transmembrane glycoprotein receptor p185^{HER2}, which has been targeted by the humanized monoclonal antibody trastuzumab (Herceptin). *HER2* is amplified and overexpressed in approximately 25% of breast cancer patients and is associated with an aggressive clinical course and poor prognosis. HER2 protein overexpression without gene amplification happens in some cases, possibly due to promoter activation and/or protein stabilization. HER2 overexpression stimulates cell growth in *p53*-mutated cells while it inhibits cell proliferation in those with wild-type *p53*. The molecular mechanisms for these differential responses have recently been clarified: the *Dmp1* promoter was activated by HER2/neu through the PI3K-Akt-NF-κB pathway, which in turn stimulated *Arf* transcription and p53 activation to prevent tumorigenesis. Conversely HER2 simply stimulate cell proliferation in cells that lack *Dmp1*, *Arf*, or *p53* (Taneja *et. al.*, 2010).

HER2 receptor overexpression has been reported in 11% to 32% of NSCLC tumors, with gene amplification found in 2%-23% of cases (Hirsch *et al.*, 2009; Swanton *et al.*, 2006). High-level ERBB2 amplification occurs in a small fraction of lung cancers with a strong propensity to high-grade adenocarcinomas (Grob *et al.*, 2012). The frequency of *HER2* amplification in NSCLC and the widespread availability of HER2 fluorescence *in situ* hybridization analysis may justify a study of trastuzumab monotherapy in NSCLC cases. However, sensitivity to HER2-directed therapies is complex and involves expression not only of HER2, but also of other EGFR family members (HER1, HER2, and HER4), their ligands, and molecules that influence pathway activity (Swanton *et al.*, 2006). The role played by HER2 as a heterodimerization partner for other EGFR family members makes HER2 an attractive target regardless of receptor overexpression in lung cancer. However, targeted therapies in patients overexpressing HER2 have proven less successful in clinical trials for NSCLC. One reason to explain the failure is intratumoral heterogeneity of *ERBB2* amplification, which was found in 4 of 10 cases (Grob *et al.*, 2012). Of note, this heterogeneity is rare in breast cancer that responds relatively well to anti-HER2 therapy. Laboratory data indicate that forced expression of HER2 in a NSCLC line increases sensitivity to gefitinib. They speculated that this may result from the gefitinib-mediated inhibition of HER2/HER3 heterodimerization and HER3 phosphorylation. It might thus be expected that combinatorial approaches, such as EGFR inhibition (by gefitinib) together with HER2 dimerization blockade (by pertuzumab) may be even more effective. Preclinical data indicate this may be the case, with the combination of erlotinib and pertuzumab promoting more than additive antitumor activity in the NSCLC (Swanton *et al.*, 2006).

While HER2 is overexpressed in about 20% of lung cancers, mutations in HER2 also occur in about 2-3% of cases. HER2 mutations typically occur in adenocarcinomas and are more frequent in women and never-smokers (Pinder, 2011). Mutations in HER2 lead to constitutive activation of the HER2 receptor, similar to the situation with EGFR. In good contrast to what we experienced in breast cancer, early clinical trials of Herceptin combined with chemotherapy in lung cancer patients with HER2 overexpression did not show a benefit for patients. However, there are case reports of lung cancer with HER2 mutations who have responded well to treatment with Herceptin plus chemotherapy. For instance, BIBW2992 (a small molecule inhibitor of EGFR and HER2) has shown evidence of activity in lung cancer patients with HER2 mutations. Most of the patients described had cancers that had shown resistance to chemotherapy and/or EGFR inhibitors. More patients with SCLC should be screened for HER2 mutations since the number of patients described to date is too small to draw any definitive conclusions (Pinder, 2011).

4.6. Cyclin D1 and lung cancer

The development of human lung carcinogenesis is very complex. Several oncogenes involved in this process have been identified, one of which is cyclin D1 (Meuwissen & Berns, 2005). Cyclin D1 is a crucial regulator in mammalian cell cycle, which drives cells to enter S phase by binding and activating CDK4/6. The cyclin D1/CDK4 complex phosphorylates the retinoblastoma protein (pRb), which releases E2F transcriptional factors from pRb constraint. The E2Fs can then activate genes that are required for the cell to enter S phase (Sherr, 1996, 2004). Cyclin D1 overexpression results in deregulation of phosphorylation of pRB, which can cause loss of growth control. In fact, Cyclin D1 gene and protein products are frequently overexpressed in a wide rang of cancers. In NSCLC, the *CCND1* locus at 11q13 is amplified in up to 32% of cases, and its protein is expressed at high level in average of 45% of all cases (Gautschi *et al.*, 2007).

The ability of cyclin D1 to cause malignant transformation has been demonstrated in breast cancer transgenic mice model, in which *MMTV-Cyclin D1* transgenic mice developed mammary AdCA (Wang *et al.*, 1994). Just like in breast cancer, *CCND1* is often found amplified and overexpressed in NSCLC patients. It has been shown that cyclin D1 overexpression is a marker for an increased risk of upper aerodigestive tract premalignant lesions for progressing to cancer (Kim *et al.*, 2011). A polymorphism, G/A870, has been identified in the *CCND1* gene and it results in an aberrantly spliced protein (Cyclin D1b) lacking the Thr-286 phosphorylation site necessary for nuclear export (Diehl *et al.*, 1997). It has been shown that the *MMTV-D1T286A* (analogous to Cyclin D1b in humans) mice developed mammary AdCAs at an increased rate relative to *MMTV-D1* mice. Even though cyclin D1b was detected in all NSCLC samples, and the G/A870 polymorphism in *CCND1* gene is predictive of the risk of lung malignancy (Gautschi *et al.*, 2007), its impact on lung carcinogenesis has never been investigated. Thus creation of mouse models for aberrant cyclin D1 expression in lung epithelial tissue is needed to test whether it is a key factor in the development of lung carcinogenesis.

Cancer chemoprevention uses dietary or pharmaceutical agents to suppress or prevent carcinogenic progression to invasive cancer. In a recent study, it was shown that a combination of retinoid bexarotene and EGFR inhibitor erlotinib can suppress lung carcinogenesis in transgenic lung cancer cells as well as NSCLC patients in both early and advanced stages. Bexarotene can induce the proteasomal degradation of cyclin D1 and erlotinib can act as an inhibitor of EGFR which represses transcription of cyclin D1 (Kim *et al.*, 2011). This finding implicates cyclin D1 as a chemopreventive target and the combination of bexarotene and erlotinib is an attractive candidate for lung cancer chemoprevention (Dragnev *et al.*, 2011). Before using this regimen in clinical lung cancer chemoprevention, its activity should first be tested in clinically predictive cyclin D1 mouse lung cancer models.

4.7. PTEN and lung cancer

Since expression of phosphatase and tensin homologue deleted from chromosome 10 (PTEN; reviewed in Inoue *et al.*, 2012) is often down regulated in NSCLC, several mice models have been generated in which *Pten* was inactivated in the bronchial epithelium (Yanagi *et al.*, 2007; Iwanaga *et al.*, 2008). *PTEN* is a tumor suppressor gene that acts by blocking the PI3K dependent activation of serine-threonine kinase Akt (Inoue *et al.*, 2012). Since $Pten^{-/-}$ mice are embryonic lethal, one had to make use of floxed *Pten* alleles ($Pten^{flox/flox}$), combined with *CCSP-Cre* transgene, targeting *Pten* deletion into bronchial epithelial cells. However, these $Pten^{flox/flox}$;*CCSP-Cre* mice did not show any aberrant pulmonary development or phenotypic abnormalities even when mice were followed for more than 12 months (Iwanaga *et al.*, 2008). This changed dramatically when the $Pten^{flox/flox}$;*CCSP-Cre* alleles were crossed with $LSLKras^{G12D}$. Lung tumor development was markedly accelerated compared in $Pten^{-/-}$;$Kras^{G12D}$ mice to that of single $LSLKras^{G12D}$ mice. *Pten*-deficient, *Kras* mutant tumors were often of the more advanced AdCA with higher vascularity (Iwanaga *et al.*, 2008), suggesting that *Pten*-loss cooperates with *Kras* mutations in NSCLC. Contrary to these results were the findings of another study in which *Pten*-inactivation was targeted in bronchioalveolar epithelium with *SPC-rtTA;tetO*$_7$*-Cre* (Yanagi *et al.*, 2007). When dox was applied *in utero* at E10-16 during embryogenesis, most mice died post-natally from hypoxia. Their lungs showed an impaired alveolar epithelial cell differentiation with an overall lung epithelial cell hyperplasia. The few surviving mice developed spontaneous lung AdCAs. Post-natal dox application during P21-27 resulted in a mild bronchiolar and alveolar cell hyperplasia and increased cell size but no lethality. A majority of these animals developed AdCAs in comparison to WT controls. Prior addition of urethane induced an even higher amount of AdCAs. Interestingly, most $Pten^{-/-}$ AdCAs (33%), with or without urethane addition, showed spontaneous *Kras* mutations. The latter observation again indicates the importance of Kras activity in cooperating with *Pten*-loss during NSCLC development.

4.8. LKB1 and lung cancer – A novel player

Mutations in liver kinase B1 (*LKB1*) are found in Peutz–Jeghers syndrome (PJS) patients and are characterized by intestinal polyps (hamartoma) and increased incidence of epithelial tumors, such as hamartomatous polyps in the gastrointestinal tract, as well as breast, colorectal, and thyroid cancers (Giardiello *et al.*, 2000). It is a serine threonine kinase also known as *STK11* (Sanchez-Cespedes *et al.*, 2002). LKB1 is a primary upstream kinase of adenine monophosphate-activated protein kinase (AMPK), a necessary element in cell metabolism that is required for maintaining energy homeostasis. It is now clear that LKB1 exerts its growth suppressing effects by activating a group of other ~14 kinases, creating a group of AMPK and AMPK-related kinases. Activation of AMPK by LKB1 suppresses cell growth and proliferation when energy and nutrient levels are low. The *LKB1* gene has been implicated in the regulation of multiple biological processes, signaling pathways (Wei *et al.*, 2005), and tumorigenesis. It has been reported that LKB1 directly activates AMP-activated kinase and regulates apoptosis in response to energy stress (Shaw *et al.*, 2004).

A large fraction of NSCLC cells have germ-line mutations and impaired expression of *LKB1*. LOH for *LKB1* has been reported in more than 50% in lung cancer (Makowski & Hayes, 2008) and thus *LKB1* inactivation is a common event for NSCLC (Sanchez-Cespedes *et al.*, 2002, Sanchez-Cespedes, 2007). The highest numbers of mutations were found in AdCAs, especially in those with *KRAS* mutations (Matsumoto *et al.*, 2007; Sanchez-Cespedes, 2007). *LKB1* inactivation cooperates with *KRAS* activation, suggesting a role for LKB1 as an active repressor of the KRAS downstream pathway (Ji *et al.*, 2007). $Lkb1^{flox/flox}$;$LSLKras^{G12D}$ mice showed a broad spectrum of NSCLCs: the majority of lung tumors were AdCAs, but SqCLCs and large cell carcinoma (LCLC) also occurred. Conversely, no SqCLC or LCLC was detected in $p53^{flox/flox}$;$LSLKras^{G12D}$ and $(Ink4a/Arf)^{flox/flox}$;$LSLKras^{G12D}$ mice. Furthermore, 61% of AdCA in $Lkb1^{flox/flox}$;$LSLKras^{G12D}$ mice developed metastases, but none found for SqCLC and LCLC. These results show that *LKB1*-loss permits squamous differentiation and facilitates metastases, but these two are independent events. AdCA from $Lkb1^{flox/flox}$;$LSLKras^{G12D}$ mice had reduced pAMPK (phosphorylated, adenosyl monophosphate-activated protein kinase) and pACCA (phosphorylated, acetyl-CoA carboxylase α-subunit) levels and activated mTOR pathway. It is probable that *LKB1*-loss influences differentiation of NSCLC into subtypes by affecting discrete pathways (Shah *et al.*, 2008). A large panel of human NSCLC showed *LKB1* mutations in AdCA (34%), SqCLC (19%), and LCC (16%) (Ji *et al.*, 2007). Simultaneous mutations in *p53* and *LKB1* suggest non-overlapping roles in NSCLC. Moreover, reconstitution of LKB1 in human NSCLC cell lines showed anti-tumor effects independent of their *p53* or *INK4A/ARF* status (Ji *et al.*, 2007). Finally, loss of LKB1 expression in alveolar adenomatous hyperplasia, precursor lesion for AdCA, suggests an early role of *LKB1*-inactivation during AdCA development (Ghaffar *et al.*, 2003).

The same group conducted a mouse trial that mirrors a human clinical trial in patients with KRAS-mutant lung cancers (Chen *et al.*, 2012). They demonstrated that simultaneous loss of either *p53* or *Lkb1*, strikingly weakened the response of *Kras*-mutant cancers to single therapy by docetaxel. Addition of selumetinib provided substantial benefit for mice with lung cancer caused by *Kras* and *Kras* and *p53* mutations, but not in mice with *Kras* and *Lkb1* mutations (Chen *et al.*, 2012). Thus synchronous 'clinical' trials performed in mice, not only will be useful to anticipate the results of ongoing human clinical trials, but also to generate clinically-relevant hypotheses that will affect the analysis and design of human studies.

4.9. miRNAs and lung cancer

Not only might genetic mutations in oncogenes and tumor suppressor genes affect their target gene expression during lung tumorigenesis, but also microRNAs (miRNAs) can also perform similar roles. microRNAs are evolutionarily conserved, endogenous, non-protein coding, 20–23 nucleotide, single-stranded RNAs that negatively regulate gene expression in a sequence-specific manner. In order to become active, small interfering RNA (siRNA) must undergo catalytic cleavage by the RNase DICER1. In human lung cancer, increased activities of DICER1 and variant regulations of miRNA clusters have been observed. For the latter, a frequent down regulation of the *let-7* miRNA family as well as an upregulation of *miR-17-92* have been reported (Hayashita *et al.*, 2005). *miR-17-92* encodes a cluster of seven miRNAs transcribed as single primary transcript. To date, functional analyses of *Dicer1* and *let-7* have been performed in the background *Kras*-induced NSCLC models. A conditional deletion of *Dicer1* in the background of *LSLKras*^{G12D};*Dicer1*$^{flox/flox}$ mice let to a marked increase of tumor development (Kumar *et al.*, 2007). However, since the 3′ UTR region of *Kras* transcripts has been shown to be a direct target of *let-7* (Johnson *et al.*, 2005), it has become very tempting to increase *let-7* expression in *Kras*^{G12D} lung tumors. *let-7* inhibits the growth of multiple human lung cancer cell lines in culture, as well as the growth of lung cancer cell xenografts *in vivo*. Intranasal application of both adenoviral (Esquela-Kerscher *et al.*, 2008) and lentiviral (Kumar *et al.*, 2008) *let-7* miRNA caused a significant decrease of *Kras*^{G12D};*p53*$^{-/-}$ lung tumors. These findings provide direct evidence that *let-7* acts as a tumor suppressor gene in the lung and indicate that this miRNA might be useful as a novel therapeutic agent in lung cancer.

A large scale survey conducted by a different group to determine the miRNA signature of >500 lung, breast, stomach, prostate, colon, and pancreatic cancers and their normal adjacent tissue revealed that *miR-21* was the only miRNA up-regulated in all these tumors (Volinia *et al.*, 2006). Functional studies in cancer cell lines suggest that *miR-21* has oncogenic activity. Knockdown of *miR-21* in cultured glioblastoma cells activated caspases leading to apoptotic cell death, suggesting *miR-21* is an anti-apoptotic factor (Chan *et al.*, 2005). In MCF-7 cells, *miR-21* knock-down resulted in suppression of cell growth both *in vitro* and *in vivo* (Si *et al.*, 2007). Knock-down of *miR-21* in the breast cancer cells reduced invasion and metastasis (Zhu *et al.*, 2008). Targeted deletion of *miR-21* colon cancer cells resulted in tumorigenesis through compromising cell cycle progression and DNA damage-induced checkpoint function by targeting *Cdc25a* (Wang *et al.*, 2009). *miR-21* expression is increased and predicts poor survival in NSCLC. Hatley *et al.* used transgenic mice with loss-of-function and gain-of-function *miR-21* alleles combined with a model of NSCLC (*K-ras*^{LA2}) to determine the role of *miR-21* in lung cancer (Hatley *et al.*, 2010). They showed that overexpression of *miR-21* enhances lung tumorigenesis and that genetic deletion of *miR-21* protects against tumor formation. *miR-21* drives tumorigenesis through inhibition of negative regulators of the Ras/MEK/ERK pathway and inhibition of apoptosis (Hatley *et al.*, 2010). These studies indicate that knocking-down of *miR-21* expression in cancer cells results in phenotypes important for tumor biology.

Hennessey *et al.* (2012) conducted Phase I/II biomarker study to examine the feasibility of using serum miRNA as biomarkers for NSCLC. Examination of miRNA expression levels in serum from a multi-institutional cohort of 50 subjects (30 NSCLC patients and 20 healthy controls) identified differentially expressed miRNAs. They found that 140 candidate miRNA pairs distinguished NSCLC from healthy controls with a sensitivity and specificity of at least 80% each. Several miRNA pairs involving miRNAs-106a, miR-15b, miR-27b, miR-142-3p, miR-26b, miR-182, 126#, let7g, let-7i (described above) and miR-30e-5p exhibited a negative predictive value and a positive predictive value of 100%. Notably, a combination of two differentially expressed miRNAs *miR-15b* and *miR-27b*, was able to discriminate NSCLC from healthy volunteers with high sensitivity, specificity (Hennessey *et al.*, 2012). Upon further testing on additional 130 subjects, this miRNA pair predicted NSCLC with a specificity of 84%, sensitivity of 100%. These data provide evidence that serum miRNAs have the potential to be sensitive, cost-effective biomarkers for the early detection of NSCLC.

5. Mouse models for squamous cell lung cancer (SqCLC)

So far genomic alterations in SqCLC have not been comprehensively characterized. The Cancer Genome Atlas group recently profiled 178 lung squamous cell carcinomas to provide a comprehensive view of genomic and epigenomic alterations (Hammerman *et al.*, 2012). They showed that the SqCLC is characterized by hundreds of exonic mutations, genomic re-arrangements, and gene copy number alterations. In addition to *TP53* mutations found in nearly all specimens, loss-of-function mutations were found in the *HLA-A* class I gene. In addition, *Nuclear factor (erythroid-derived 2)-like 2*, *Kelch-like ECH-associated protein 1*, *Squamous differentiation*, and *Phosphatidylinositol-3-OH kinase pathway* genes were frequently altered. *CDKN2A* and *RB1* genes were inactivated in as many as 72% of SqCLC cases. This comprehensive study identified a potential therapeutic target in most tumors, offering new avenues of investigation for the treatment of human SqCLC (Hammerman *et al.*, 2012).

Although squamous cell carcinoma is a common type of lung cancer causing nearly 400,000 deaths per year worldwide, there is no established gene-engineered mouse model for squamous cell carcinoma of the lung. Human lung SqCLC is closely linked with smoking and shows a distinct order of pre-malignant changes in the bronchial epithelium from hyperplasia, metaplasia, dysplasia and carcinoma *in situ* to invasive and metastatic SqCLC (Brambilla *et al.*, 2000). A better understanding of the cell of origin that give rise to SqCLC and identification of unique genetic alterations that are specific to lung squamous cell carcinoma as reported by the comprehensive study might help to create SqCLC mouse models. One important issue that should be taken into account is that normal human or mouse lungs do not contain squamous epithelium. Mice do not smoke, so only under pathological conditions does squamous metaplasia accompanied by high expression levels of keratins occur in the airway epithelium (Wistuba *et al.*, 2002, 2003). Only a few mouse models reported the onset of SqCLC, mostly after carcinogen application. For instance, intratracheal intubation of methyl carbamate (Jetten *et al.*, 1992) or extensive topical application of *N*-nitroso-compounds (Nettesheim *et al.*, 1971; Rehm *et al.*, 1991) caused SqCLC in mice. Wang *et al.* (2004) treated eight different inbred strains of mice with N-nitroso-tris-chloroethylurea by skin painting and found that this chemical induced SqCLCs in five strains (SWR, Swiss, A/J, BALB/c, and FVB), but not in the others (AKR, 129/svJ, and C57BL/6). Besides, specific loci for SqCLC susceptibility have been identified through linkage analyses in several mice strains (Wang *et al.*, 2004), using 6,128 markers in publically available databases. Three markers (*D1Mit169*, *D3Mit178*, and *D18Mit91*) were found significantly associated with susceptibility to SqCLC. Interestingly, none of these sites overlapped with the major susceptibility loci associated with lung adenoma/adenocarcinomas in mice indicating that different

http://dx.doi.org/10.5772/53721

sets of genes are responsible for SqCLC and AdCA. Their model can be used in determining genetic modifiers that contribute to susceptibility or resistance to SqCLC development.

The other group tried to induce SqCLC through constitutive expression of human K14 by creating *CC10-hK14* mice (Dakir *et al.*, 2008). Although hK14 is highly expressed in bronchial epithelium, only precursor lesions varying from hyperplasia to squamous metaplasia were observed (Dakir *et al.*, 2008). Clearly, the increased K14 expression and onset of squamous cell metaplasia alone was not sufficient to generate fully developed SqCLC. As far as transgenic/knockout mice models are concerned, only the *LSLKras*^{G12D};*Lkb1*$^{flox/flox}$ somatic mouse model has been able to generate advanced SqCLC. By using a somatically activatable mutant *Kras*-driven model of mouse lung cancer (*K-ras*^{LA}), Ji *et al.* (2007) compared the role of Lkb1 to other tumor suppressors in lung cancer. Although *Kras* mutation cooperated with loss of *p53* or *Ink4a/Arf* in this system, the strongest cooperation was seen with homozygous inactivation of *Lkb1*. *Lkb1*-deficient tumors demonstrated shorter latency, an expanded histological spectrum (adeno-, squamous, and large-cell carcinoma) and more frequent metastasis as compared to tumors lacking *p53* or *Ink4a/Arf*. Interestingly up to 60% of *Lkb1* deficient lung tumors had squamous or mixed squamous histology (Ji *et al.*, 2007), which has not been reported in other mouse lung cancer models. Pulmonary tumorigenesis was also accelerated by hemizygous inactivation of *Lkb1*, confirming its haplo-insufficiency. Consistent with these findings, inactivation of *LKB1* was found in 34% and 19% of 144 human lung adenocarcinomas and squamous cell carcinomas, respectively. They also identified a variety of metastasis-promoting genes, such as *NEDD9*, *VEGFC* and *CD24*, as targets of LKB1 repression in lung cancer. These studies established LKB1 as a critical barrier to prevent lung carcinogenesis, controlling initiation, differentiation and metastasis (Ji *et al.*, 2007).

6. Clinical implications and future directions for mouse lung cancer models

Xenograft models where manipulated human lung cancer cell lines are subcutaneously injected into nude mice have been extensively used for pre-clinical testing of novel drugs for lung cancer. The major issue for this approach is that lung cancer cell lines have already been adapted for long-term culture in a plastic dish with artificial medium and acquired stem-cell like phenotypes, and thus are not suitable for models of primary human lung cancer obtained by surgical resection. The more preferred method, however, have been orthotopical transplantation of human lung tumor cells in their lung cavity. To date, the results have shown that xenograft models do not accurately predict the clinical efficacy of anti-tumor drugs. Therefore, a question arises as to whether spontaneous and/or genetically-engineered mouse models for lung cancer would be more useful as tools for pre-clinical drug tests. It is obvious that there are differences in the lung anatomy and physiology between mice and humans, but some of the mouse models that we have described have a striking histological similarity, with an analogous genetic signature to that of human NSCLC. Importantly, genetically-engineered mouse model-derived tumors develop in an innate immune environment and, therefore, have all the tumor-stromal interactions, such as angiogenesis and degradation of the tissue matrix.

We have described two models for NSCLC in which either the continuous oncogenic activity of Kras (Fisher *et al*, 2001) or EGFR (Politi *et al*, 2006) are prerequisites of tumor maintenance since lung tumors underwent spontaneous regression with disappearance of the oncogene by dox withdrawal. This not only shows that tumor growth critically depends on the initiating active oncogenic pathways, but it also stresses the usefulness of these oncogenic pathways as therapeutic targets. Direct tumor intervention studies with tyrosine kinase inhibitors against EGFR mutations proved to be highly effective in several *hEGFR*-transgenic mouse models. TKIs such as gefitinib, erlotinib, and HKI-272 led to complete tumor regression (Politi *et al.*, 2006; Ji *et al.*, 2006a,b). In addition, treatment of lung cancer with humanized anti-hEGFR antibody (cetuximab) caused a significant tumor regression (Ji *et al.*, 2006a). Further studies will be needed to investigate the signaling cascades that determine the sensitivity and resistance to EGFR-related tyrosine kinase interventions.

Other mouse models for NSCLC have also been used for targeted therapies. First, dox-induced overexpression of the PI3K p110α catalytic subunit PIK3CA, mutated in its kinase domain (H1047R) in *CCSP-rtTA;tetO$_7$-PIK3CA(H1047R)* mice, induces adenocarcinomas (Engelman *et al.*, 2008). Treatment of these lung tumors with NVP-BEZ235, a dual pan-PI3K and mammalian target of rapamycin (mTOR) inhibitor, caused a marked lung tumor regression. Interestingly, when this single agent NVP6-BEZ235 was tested on lung tumors in *CCSP-rtTA;tetO$_7$-Kras^{G12D}* mice, no regression was observed. However, when NVP-BEZ235 was combined with MEK inhibitor ARRY-142886, significant regression of *Kras^{G12D}* tumors occurred (Engelman *et al.*, 2008). Thus, two major RAS downstream effector pathways needed to be inactivated to get an irreversible regression in Ras mutated NSCLC.

Although *K-RAS* is mutated in ~30% of human NSCLC, direct targeting of RAS has been unsuccessful for lung cancer therapy. Many small molecules against Ras functions have been tested and farnesyl transferase inhibitors are the most marked examples of these failed attempts (Mahgoub *et al.*, 1999; Omer *et al.*, 2000). Recent results with lung cancer mouse models strongly suggest that KRAS4A, and not KRAS4B is driving the onset of NSCLC. An explanation for this failure can thus be attributed to the fact that only KRAS4B is farnesylated, but not its isoform KRAS4A. Although we still have to study if KRAS4A is important in the pathogenesis of human NSCLC, we can imagine the importance of *Kras* mouse models in testing functional inhibitiors for KRAS4A (To *et al.*, 2008).

The use of optimized, genetically-modified mouse models for lung cancer for therapy research necessitates sophisticated non-invasive tools to follow tumor development and response to therapy *in vivo*. Measurement of tumor size as a function of time is the most obvious way of doing this and existing techniques such as computed-tomography imaging or magnetic resonance imaging for small animals are now in use (Engelman *et al.*, 2008; Politi *et al.*, 2006). However, these techniques are time-consuming and expensive, making them less suitable for large number of animals. Other techniques, such as fluorescence imaging and bioluminescence, can be used for measuring gene expression or tumor growth *in vivo*

(Contag *et al.*, 2000; Hadjantonakis *et al.*, 2003). In case of latter studies, transgenic expression of luciferase allows accurate longitudinal monitoring and good quantification of tumor burden as has been shown in the *LSL Kras* lung tumor model (Jackson *et al.*, 2001). These novel imaging techniques will greatly enhance the accuracy and reproducibility of mouse models.

Transgenic lung cancer models created by Chen *et al*. (2002) can be applied to clinics by raising Ron-specific antibodies. O'Toole *et al.* (2006) conducted an antibody phage display library to generate a human IgG1 antibody IMC-41A10 that binds with high affinity to RON and effectively blocks interaction with its ligand, macrophage-stimulating protein. They found IMC-41A10 to be a potent inhibitor of receptor and downstream signaling, cell migration, and tumorigenesis. It antagonized MSP-induced phosphorylation of RON, MAPK, and AKT in several cancer cell lines. In NCI-H292 lung cancer xenograft tumor models, IMC-41A10 inhibited tumor growth by 50% to 60% as a single agent. This antibody should be tested *in vivo* using the *SPC-RON* mice with developing lung AdCAs.

Recent strategies showed the importance of aberrant promoter methylation in lung cancer development, such a *p16*^{INK4a}, *Death-associated protein kinase 1,* and, *RAS association domain family 1A* (Shames *et al.*, 2006). Since chronic inflammations have been implicated in cancer pathogenesis (Shacter & Weitzman, 2002), altered methylation for lung surfactant proteins are good topics for future lung cancer studies; their signatures may serve as valuable markers in lung cancer detection. The lung surfactant protein (*SP*) genes, *SP-A* and *SP-D* have been identified with high throughput approach that showed an altered methylation pattern in lung cancer compared to normal lung tissue (Vaid & Floros, 2009). However, *SP-A*-deficient mice were able to survive with no apparent pathology in a sterile environment (Korfhagen et al., 1996), although their pulmonary immune responses were insufficient during immune challenge. *SP-D*-deficient mice, on the other hand, showed phenotypic abnormalities in alveolar macrophages and type II pneumocytes with increased lipid pools, indicating that *SP-D* has an important role in surfactant homeostasis (Botas et al., 1998). Paradoxically overexpression of *SP-A* and/or *SP-D* as a result of promoter hypomethylation has also been reported in lung cancer suggesting that it is critical to keep these protein levels within physiological ranges to prevent neoplastic transformation. Since the role of these lung surfactant proteins in lung carcinogenesis has never been studied *in vivo*, it will be worthwhile to cross lung surfactant-deficient mice with available transgenic/knockout strains to elucidate the roles of surfactant proteins in lung cancer initiation and development.

Acknowledgements

K. Inoue has been supported by NIH/NCI 5R01CA106314, ACS RSG-07-207-01-MGO, and by WFUCCC Director's Challenge Award #20595. D. Maglic has been supported by DOD pre-doctoral fellowship BC100907. We thank K. Klein for editorial assistance.

Author details

Kazushi Inoue[1,2,3*], Elizabeth Fry[1,2], Dejan Maglic[1,2,3] and Sinan Zhu[1,3]

*Address all correspondence to: kinoue2@triad.rr.com

*Address all correspondence to: drkazu12000@yahoo.com

1 The Department of Pathology, Wake Forest University Health Sciences, Medical Center Boulevard, Winston-Salem, NC, USA

2 The Department of Cancer Biology, Wake Forest University Health Sciences, Medical Center Boulevard, Winston-Salem, NC, USA

3 Graduate Program in Molecular Medicine, Wake Forest University Health Sciences, Medical Center Boulevard, Winston-Salem, NC, USA

References

[1] Siegel R, Naishadham D, Jemal A. Cancer statistics, 2012. *CA Cancer J Clin* 2012;62:10-29.

[2] Centers for Disease Control and Prevention (CDC). Racial/Ethnic disparities and geographic differences in lung cancer incidence --- 38 States and the District of Columbia, 1998-2006. *MMWR Morb Mortal Wkly Rep* 2010;59:1434-8.

[3] Wisnivesky JP, McGinn T, Henschke C, Hebert P, Iannuzzi MC, Halm EA. Ethnic disparities in the treatment of stage I non-small cell lung cancer. *Am J Respir Crit Care Med* 2005;171:1158-63.

[4] Swierzewski III, SJ. Lung Cancer Environmental Risk Factors. 1999. http://www.healthcommunities.com/lung-cancer/environmental.shtml

[5] Menon P. Lung Cancer: Delayed Diagnosis Among Non-Smokers. 2012. http://trialx.com/curetalk/2012/06/lung-cancer-delayed-diagnosis-among-non-smokers/

[6] Brambilla C, Fievet F, Jeanmart M, *et al*. Early detection of lung cancer: role of biomarkers. *Eur Respir J Suppl* 2003;39:36s-44s.

[7] Yeung SC, Habra MA, Thosani SN. Lung cancer-induced paraneoplastic syndromes. *Curr Opin Pulm Med* 2011;17:260-8.

[8] Moran CA. Pulmonary adenocarcinoma: The expanding spectrum of histologic variants. *Arch Pathol Lab Med* 2006;130:958-62.

[9] Schiller JH. Current standards of care in small-cell and non-small-cell lung cancer. *Oncology* 2001;61, Suppl 1:3-13.

[10] Travis WD. Pathology of lung cancer. *Clin Chest Med* 2002;23,65-81.

[11] Zochbauer-Muller S, Gazdar AF, and Minna JD. Molecular pathogenesis of lung cancer. *Ann Rev Physiol* 2002;64,681-708.

[12] Fong KM, Sekido Y, Gazdar AF, and Minna JD. Lung cancer. 9: Molecular biology of lung cancer: Clinical implications. *Thorax* 2003;58:892-900.

[13] Meuwissen R and Berns A. Mouse models for human lung cancer. *Genes Dev* 2005;19:643-64.

[14] Worden FP, Kalemkerian GP. Therapeutic advances in small cell lung cancer. *Expert Opin Investig Drugs* 2000;9:565-79.

[15] Wakamatsu N, Devereux TR, Hong HH, *et al*. Overview of the molecular carcinogenesis of mouse lung tumor models of human lung cancer. *Toxicol Pathol* 2007;35:75-80.

[16] Shimkin MB, Stoner GD. Lung tumors in mice: application to carcinogenesis bioassay. *Adv Cancer Res* 1975;21:1-58.

[17] Pfeifer GP, Denissenko MF, Olivier M, *et al*. Tobacco smoke carcinogens, DNA damage and p53 mutations in smoking-associated cancers. *Oncogene* 2002;21:7435-51.

[18] Sato M, Shames DS, Gazdar AF, *et al*. A translational view of the molecular pathogenesis of lung cancer. *J Thorac Oncol* 2007;2:327-43.

[19] Malkinson AM. Primary lung tumors in mice as an aid for understanding, preventing, and treating human AdCA of the lung. *Lung Cancer* 2001;32:265-79.

[20] DeMayo FJ, Finegold MJ, Hansen TN, *et al*. Expression of SV40 T antigen under control of rabbit uteroglobin promoter in transgenic mice. *Am J Physiol* 1991;261:L70-6.

[21] Sandmoller A, Halter R, Gomez-La-Hoz E, *et al*. The uteroglobin promoter targets expression of the SV40 T antigen to a variety of secretory epithelial cells in transgenic mice. *Oncogene* 1994;9:2805-15.

[22] Wikenheiser KA, Clark JC, Linnoila RI, *et al*. Simian virus 40 large T antigen directed by transcriptional elements of the human surfactant protein C gene produces pulmonary AdCAs in transgenic mice. *Cancer Res* 1992;52:5342-52.

[23] Wikenheiser KA, Whitsett JA. Tumor progression and cellular differentiation of pulmonary AdCAs in SV40 large T antigen transgenic mice. *Am J Respir Cell Mol Biol* 1997;16:713-23.

[24] Geick A, Redecker P, Ehrhardt A, *et al.* Uteroglobin promoter-targeted c-MYC expression in transgenic mice cause hyperplasia of Clara cells and malignant transformation of T-lymphoblasts and tubular epithelial cells. *Transgenic Res* 2001;10:501-11.

[25] Ehrhardt A, Bartels T, Geick A, Klocke R, Paul D, Halter R. Development of pulmonary bronchiolo-alveolar AdCAs in transgenic mice overexpressing murine c-myc and epidermal growth factor in alveolar type II pneumocytes. *Br J Cancer* 2001;84:813-8.

[26] Sunday ME, Haley KJ, Sikorski K, *et al*. Calcitonin driven v-Ha-ras induces multilineage pulmonary epithelial hyperplasias and neoplasms. *Oncogene* 1999;18:36-47.

[27] Mallakin A, Sugiyama T, Taneja P, *et al*. Mutually exclusive inactivation of DMP1 and ARF/p53 in lung cancer. *Cancer Cell* 2007;12:381-94.

[28] Morris GF, Hoyle GW, Athas GB, *et al*. Lung-specific expression in mice of a dominant negative mutant form of the p53 tumor suppressor protein. *J La State Med Soc* 1998;150:179-85.

[29] Tchou-Wong KM, Jiang Y, Yee H, *et al.* Lung-specific expression of dominant-negative mutant p53 in transgenic mice increases spontaneous and benzo(a)pyrene-induced lung cancer. *Am J Respir Cell Mol Biol* 2002;27:186-93.

[30] Chen YQ, Zhou YQ, Fu LH, Wang D, Wang MH. Multiple pulmonary adenomas in the lung of transgenic mice overexpressing the RON receptor tyrosine kinase. Recepteur d'origine nantais. *Carcinogenesis* 2002;23:1811-9.

[31] Sekido Y, Fong KM, Minna JD. Molecular genetics of lung cancer. *Annu Rev Med* 2003;54:73-87.

[32] Jacks T, Fazeli A, Schmitt EM, *et al*. Effects of an Rb mutation in the mouse. *Nature* 1992;359:295-300.

[33] Meuwissen R, Berns A. Mouse models for human lung cancer. *Genes Dev* 2005;19:643-64.

[34] Olive KP, Tuveson DA, Ruhe ZC, *et al*. Mutant p53 gain of function in two mouse models of Li-Fraumeni syndrome. *Cell* 2004;119:847-60.

[35] Lang GA, Iwakuma T, Suh YA, *et al*. Gain of function of a p53 hot spot mutation in a mouse model of Li-Fraumeni syndrome. *Cell* 2004;119:861-72.

[36] Smith AJ, Xian J, Richardson M, *et al*. Cre-loxP chromosome engineering of a targeted deletion in the mouse corresponding to the 3p21.3 region of homozygous loss in human tumors. *Oncogene* 2002;21:4521-9.

[37] Tommasi S, Dammann R, Zhang Z, *et al*. Tumor susceptibility of Rassf1a knockout mice. *Cancer Res* 2005;65:92–8.

[38] Zanesi N, Mancini R, Sevignani C, *et al*. Lung cancer susceptibility in Fhit-deficient mice is increased by Vhl haploinsufficiency. *Cancer Res* 2005;65:6576-82.

[39] Johnson L, Mercer K, Greenbaum D, *et al*. Somatic activation of the K-ras oncogene causes early onset lung cancer in mice. *Nature* 2001;410:1111-6.

[40] Hirai H, Sherr CJ. Interaction of D-type cyclins with a novel myb-like transcription factor, DMP1. *Mol Cell Biol* 1996;16:6457-67.

[41] Inoue K, Sherr CJ. Gene expression and cell cycle arrest mediated by transcription factor DMP1 is antagonized by D-type cyclins through a cyclin-dependent-kinase-independent mechanism. *Mol Cell Biol* 1998;18:1590-600.

[42] Inoue K, Mallakin A, and Frazier DP. Dmp1 and tumor suppression. *Oncogene* 2007;26:4329-35. Review.

[43] Sugiyama T, Frazier DP, Taneja P, *et al*. Signal transduction involving the Dmp1 transcription factor and its alteration in human cancer. *Clinical Medicine Insights: Oncology* 2008a; 2:209-19.

[44] Inoue K, Roussel MF, and Sherr CJ. Induction of ARF tumor suppressor gene expression and cell cycle arrest by transcription factor DMP1. *Proc Natl Acad Sci USA* 1999;96:3993-8.

[45] Sreeramaneni R, Chaudhry A, McMahon M, Sherr CJ, and Inoue K. Ras-Raf-Arf signaling critically depends on the Dmp1 transcription factor. *Mol Cell Biol* 2005;25:220-32.

[46] Inoue K, Wen R, Rehg JE, Adachi M, Cleveland JL, Roussel MF, and Sherr CJ. Functional loss of the ARF transcriptional activator DMP1 facilitates cell immortalization, ras transformation, and tumorigenesis. *Genes Dev* 2000;14:1797-809.

[47] Inoue K, Zindy F, Randle DH, Rehg JE, and Sherr CJ. Dmp1 is haplo-insufficient for tumor suppression and modifies the frequencies of Arf and p53 mutations in Myc-induced lymphomas. *Genes Dev* 2001;15:2934-9.

[48] Mallakin A, Sugiyama T, Taneja P, *et al*. Mutually exclusive inactivation of DMP1 and ARF/p53 in lung cancer. *Cancer Cell* 2007;12:381-94.

[49] Sugiyama T, Frazier DP, Taneja P, *et al*. The role of Dmp1 and its future in lung cancer diagnostics. *Expert Rev Mol Diagn* 2008b;8:435-48.

[50] Sweet-Cordero A, Mukherjee S, Subramanian A, *et al*. An oncogenic KRAS2 expression signature identified by cross-species gene-expression analysis. *Nat Genet* 2005;37:48-55.

[51] Jackson EL, Willis N, Mercer K, *et al*. Analysis of lung tumor initiation and progression using conditional expression of oncogenic K-ras. *Genes Dev* 2001;15:3243-8.

[52] Jackson EL, Olive KP, Tuveson DA, Bronson R, Crowley D, Brown M, and Jacks T. The differential effects of mutant p53 alleles on advanced murine lung cancer. *Cancer Res* 2005;65:10280-8.

[53] Ji H, Houghton AM, Mariani TJ, *et al*. K-ras activation generates an inflammatory response in lung tumors. *Oncogene* 2006;25:2105-12.

[54] Jonkers J, Berns A. Conditional mouse models of sporadic cancer. *Nat Rev Cancer* 2002;2:251-65.

[55] Lewandoski M. Conditional control of gene expression in the mouse. *Nat Rev Genet* 2001;2:743-55.

[56] Gossen M, Bujard H. Tight control of gene expression in mammalian cells by tet-responsive promoters. *Proc Natl Acad Sci USA* 1992;89:5547-51.

[57] Perl AK, Tichelaar JW, Whitsett JA. Conditional gene expression in the respiratory epithelium of the mouse. *Transgenic Res* 2002;11:21-9.

[58] Floyd HS, Farnsworth CL, Kock ND, *et al*. Conditional expression of the mutant Ki-rasG12C allele results in formation of benign lung adenomas: development of a novel mouse lung tumor model. *Carcinogenesis* 2005;26:2196-206.

[59] Tichelaar JW, Lu W, Whitsett JA. Conditional expression of fibroblast growth factor-7 in the developing and mature lung. *J Biol Chem* 2000;275:11858–64.

[60] Fisher GH, Wellen SL, Klimstra D, *et al*. Induction and apoptotic regression of lung adenocarcinomas by regulation of a K-Ras transgene in the presence and absence of tumor suppressor genes. *Genes Dev* 2001;15:3249-62.

[61] Dutt A, Wong KK. Novel agents in the treatment of lung cancer: advances in EGFR-targeted agents: mouse models of lung cancer. *Clin Cancer Res* 2006;12:4396s-402s.

[62] Jackson EL, Willis N, Mercer K, *et al*. Analysis of lung tumor initiation and progression using conditional expression of oncogenic K-ras. *Genes Dev* 2001;15:3243-8.

[63] Meuwissen R, Linn SC, van der Vaulk M, *et al*. Mouse model for lung tumorigenesis through Cre/lox controlled sporadic activation of the K-Ras oncogene. *Oncogene* 2001;20:6551–58.

[64] Guerra C, Mijimolle N, Dhawahir A, *et al*. Tumor induction by an endogenous K-ras oncogene is highly dependent on cellular context. *Cancer Cell* 2003;4:111–120.

[65] Ji H, Wang Z, Perera SA, *et al*. Mutations in BRAF and KRAS converge on activation of the mitogen-activated protein kinase pathway in lung cancer mouse models. *Cancer Res* 2007;67:4933-9.

[66] Davies H, Bignell GR, Cox C, *et al*. Mutations of the BRAF gene in human cancer. *Nature* 2002;417:949-54.

[67] Mercer KE, Pritchard CA. Raf proteins and cancer: B-Raf is identified as a mutational target. *Biochim Biophys Acta* 2003;1653:25-40. Review.

[68] Dankort D, Filenova E, Collado M, Serrano M, Jones K, McMahon M. A new mouse model to explore the initiation, progression, and therapy of BRAFV600E-induced lung tumors. *Genes Dev* 2007;21:379-84.

[69] Blasco RB, Francoz S, Santamaría D, *et al*. c-Raf, but not B-Raf, is essential for development of K-Ras oncogene-driven non-small cell lung carcinoma. *Cancer Cell* 2011;19:652-63.

[70] Shaw AT, Meissner A, Dowdle JA, *et al*. Sprouty-2 regulates oncogenic K-ras in lung development and tumorigenesis. *Genes Dev* 2007;21:694-707.

[71] Cho HC, Lai CY, Shao LE, Yu J. Identification of tumorigenic cells in Kras(G12D)-induced lung AdCA. *Cancer Res* 2011;71:7250-8.

[72] Samuels Y, Velculescu VE. Oncogenic mutations of PIK3CA in human cancers. *Cell Cycle* 2004;3:1221-4.

[73] Wojtalla A, Arcaro A. Targeting phosphoinositide 3-kinase signalling in lung cancer. *Critical Reviews in Oncology/Hematology* 2011;80:278-290.

[74] Angulo B, Suarez-Gauthier A, Lopez-Rios F, *et al*. Expression signatures in lung cancer reveal a profile for EGFR-mutant tumors and identify selective PIK3CA overexpression by gene amplification. *J Pathol* 2008;214:347-56.

[75] Engelman JA, Chen L, Tan X, *et al*. Effective use of PI3K and MEK inhibitors to treat mutant Kras G12D and PIK3CA H1047R murine lung cancers. *Nat Med* 2008;14:1351-6.

[76] Gupta S, Ramjaun AR, Haiko P, *et al*. Binding of ras to phosphoinositide 3-kinase p110alpha is required for ras-driven tumorigenesis in mice. *Cell* 2007;129:957-68.

[77] Mack NA, Whalley HJ, Castillo-Lluva S, Malliri A. The diverse roles of Rac signaling in tumorigenesis. *Cell Cycle* 2011;10:1571-81.

[78] Kissil JL, Walmsley MJ, Hanlon L, *et al*. Requirement for Rac1 in a K-ras induced lung cancer in the mouse. *Cancer Res* 2007;67:8089-94.

[79] Stella GM, Luisetti M, Inghilleri S, *et al*. Targeting EGFR in non-small-cell lung cancer: Lessons, experiences, strategies. *Resp Med* 2012;106,173-83.

[80] Lynch TJ, Bell DW, Sordella R, *et al*. Activating mutations in the epidermal growth factor receptor underlying responsiveness of non-small-cell lung cancer to gefitinib. *N Engl J Med* 2004;350:2129-39.

[81] Soria J-C, Mok TS, Cappuzzo F, *et al*. EGFR-mutated oncogene-addicted non-small cell lung cancer: Current trends and future prospects. *Cancer Treat Rev* 2012;38,416-30.

[82] Ji H, Zhao X, Yuza Y, *et al*. Epidermal growth factor receptor variant III mutations in lung tumorigenesis and sensitivity to tyrosine kinase inhibitors. *Proc Natl Acad Sci USA*. 2006a;103:7817-22. Epub 2006 May 3.

[83] Ji H, Li D, Chen L, *et al*. The impact of human EGFR kinase domain mutations on lung tumorigenesis and in vivo sensitivity to EGFR-targeted therapies. *Cancer Cell* 2006b;9:485-95.

[84] Politi K, Zakowski MF, Fan PD, *et al*. Lung adenocarcinomas induced in mice by mutant EGF receptors found in human lung cancers respond to a tyrosine kinase inhibitor or to down-regulation of the receptors. *Genes Dev* 2006;20:1496-510.

[85] Li D, Shimamura T, Ji H, Chen L *et al*. Bronchial and Peripheral Murine Lung Carcinomas Induced by T790M-L858R Mutant EGFR Respond to HKI-272 and Rapamycin Combination Therapy. *Cancer Cell* 2007;12:81-93.

[86] Hu Y, Bandla S, Godfrey TE, Tan D, *et al*. HER2 amplification, overexpression and score criteria in esophageal adenocarcinoma. *Mod Pathol* 2011;24:899-907.

[87] Taneja P, Maglic D, Kai F, *et al*. Critical role of Dmp1 in HER2/neu-p53 signaling and breast carcinogenesis. *Cancer Res* 70: 9084-94, 2010.

[88] Hirsch FR, Varella-Garcia M, Cappuzzo F. Predictive value of EGFR and HER2 overexpression in advanced non-small-cell lung cancer. *Oncogene* 2009;28 Suppl 1:S32-7.

[89] Swanton C, Futreal A, Eisen T. Her2-targeted therapies in non-small cell lung cancer. *Clin Cancer Res* 2006;12(14 Pt 2):4377s-83s.

[90] Grob TJ, Kannengiesser I, Tsourlakis MC, *et al*. Heterogeneity of ERBB2 amplification in adenocarcinoma, squamous cell carcinoma and large cell undifferentiated carcinoma of the lung. *Mod Pathol* 2012 Aug 17. doi: 10.1038/modpathol.2012.125. [Epub ahead of print]

[91] Pinder. Lesser Known Lung Cancer Mutations Part 1: HER2, a promising therapeutic target? http://cancergrace.org/lung/2011/03/19/her2-by-m/

[92] Meuwissen R and Berns A. Mouse models for human lung cancer. *Genes Dev* 2005;19,643-64.

[93] Sherr CJ. Cancer cell cycles. *Science* 1996;274:1672-7. Review.

[94] Sherr CJ. Principles of tumor suppression. *Cell* 2004;116:235-46. Review.

[95] Jiang W, Kahn SM, Zhou P, *et al*. Overexpression of cyclin D1 in rat fibroblasts causes abnormalities in growth control, cell cycle progression and gene expression. *Oncogene* 1993;8:3447-57.

[96] Gautschi O, Ratschiller D, Gugger M, Betticher DC, Heighway J. Cyclin D1 in non-small cell lung cancer: A key driver of malignant transformation. *Lung Cancer* 2007;55:1-14.

[97] Wang TC, Cardiff RD, Zukerberg L, *et al*. Mammary hyperplasia and carcinoma in MMTV-cyclin D1 transgenic mice. *Nature* 1994 ;369:669-71.

[98] Kim ES, Lee JJ, Wistuba II. Cotargeting Cyclin D1 Starts a New Chapter in Lung Cancer Prevention and Therapy. *Cancer Prevention Research* 2011;4:779-82.

[99] Diehl JA, Zindy F, Sherr CJ. Inhibition of cyclin D1 phosphorylation on threonine-286 prevents its rapid degradation via the ubiquitin-proteasome pathway. *Genes Dev* 1997;11:957-72.

[100] Dragnev KH, Ma T, Cyrus J, *et al*. Bexarotene Plus Erlotinib Suppress Lung Carcinogenesis Independent of KRAS Mutations in Two Clinical Trials and Transgenic Models. *Cancer Prev Res* 2011;4:818-28.

[101] Yanagi S, Kishimoto H, Kawahara K, *et al*. Pten controls lung morphogenesis, bronchioalveolar stem cells, and onset of lung adenocarcinomas in mice. *J Clin Invest* 2007;117:2929–40.

[102] Inoue K, Kulik G, Fry EA, Zhu S, and Maglic D. Recent progress in mouse models for tumor suppressor genes and its implications in human cancer (review). *Clinical Medicine Insights: Oncology*, submitted (2012).

[103] Iwanaga K, Yang Y, Raso MG, *et al*. Pten inactivation accelerates oncogenic K-ras-initiated tumorigenesis in a mouse model of lung cancer. *Cancer Res* 2008;68:1119-27.

[104] Yanagi S, Kishimoto H, Kawahara K, *et al*. Pten controls lung morphogenesis, bronchioalveolar stem cells, and onset of lung adenocarcinomas in mice. *J Clin Invest* 2007;117:2929–40.

[105] Iwanaga K, Yang Y, Raso MG, *et al*. Pten inactivation accelerates oncogenic K-ras-initiated tumorigenesis in a mouse model of lung cancer. *Cancer Res* 2008;68:1119-27.

[106] Giardiello FM, Brensinger JD, Tersmette AC, *et al*. Very high risk of cancer in familial Peutz-Jeghers syndrome. *Gastroenterology* 2000;119:1447–53.

[107] Sanchez-Cespedes M, Parrella P, Esteller M, *et al*. Inactivation of LKB1/STK11 is a common event in AdCAs of the lung. *Cancer Res* 2002;62:3659–62.

[108] Wei C, Amos CI, Stephens LC, *et al*. Mutation of Lkb1 and p53 genes exert a cooperative effect on tumorigenesis. *Cancer Res* 2005;65:11297-303.

[109] Shaw RJ, Kosmatka M, Bardeesy N, *et a*l. The tumor suppressor LKB1 kinase directly activates AMP-activated kinase and regulates apoptosis in response to energy stress. *Proc Natl Acad Sci USA* 2004;101:3329-35.

[110] Makowski L, Hayes DN. Role of LKB1 in lung cancer development. *Br J Cancer* 2008;99:683-8.

[111] Sanchez-Cespedes M. A role for LKB1 gene in human cancer beyond the Peutz-Jeghers syndrome. *Oncogene* 2007;26:7825-32.

[112] Matsumoto S, Iwakawa R, Takahashi K, *et al*. Prevalence and specificity of LKB1 genetic alterations in lung cancers. *Oncogene* 2007;26:5911-8.

[113] Ji H, Ramsey MR, Hayes DN, *et al*. LKB1 modulates lung cancer differentiation and metastasis. *Nature* 2007;448:807-10.

[114] Shah U, Sharpless NE, Hayes DN. LKB1 and lung cancer: more than the usual suspects. *Cancer Res* 2008;68:3562-65.

[115] Ghaffar H, Sahin F, Sanchez-Cepedes M, *et al*. LKB1 protein expression in the evolution of glandular neoplasia of the lung. *Clin Cancer Res* 2003;9:2998-3003.

[116] Chen Z, Cheng K, Walton Z, *et al*. A murine lung cancer co-clinical trial identifies genetic modifiers of therapeutic response. *Nature* 2012;483:613-7.

[117] Hayashita Y, Osada H, Tatematsu Y, *et al*. A polycistronic microRNA cluster, miR-17-92, is overexpressed in human lung cancers and enhances cell proliferation. *Cancer Res* 2005;65:9628-32.

[118] Kumar MS, Lu J, Mercer KL, *et al*. Impaired microRNA processing enhances cellular transformation and tumorigenesis. *Nat Genet* 2007;39:673-7.

[119] Johnson SM, Grosshans H, Shingara J, *et al*. RAS is regulated by the let-7 microRNA family. *Cell* 2005;120:635-47.

[120] Esquela-Kerscher A, Trang P, Wiggins JF, *et al*. The let-7 microRNA reduces tumor growth in mouse models of lung cancer. *Cell Cycle* 2008;7:759-64.

[121] Kumar MS, Erkeland SJ, Pester RE, *et al*. Suppression of non-small cell lung tumor development by the let-7 microRNA family. *Proc Natl Acad Sci USA* 2008;105:3903-8.

[122] Volinia S, Calin GA, Liu CG, *et al*. A microRNA expression signature of human solid tumors defines cancer gene targets. *Proc Natl Acad Sci USA* 2006;103:2257-61.

[123] Chan JA, Krichevsky AM, Kosik KS. MicroRNA-21 is an antiapoptotic factor in human glioblastoma cells. *Cancer Res* 2005;65:6029-33.

[124] Si ML, Zhu S, Wu H, Lu Z, Wu F, Mo YY. miR-21-mediated tumor growth. *Oncogene* 2007;26:2799-803.

[125] Zhu S, Wu H, Wu F, Nie D, Sheng S, Mo YY. MicroRNA-21 targets tumor suppressor genes in invasion and metastasis. *Cell Res* 2008;18:350-9.

[126] Wang P, Zou F, Zhang X, *et al*. microRNA-21 negatively regulates Cdc25A and cell cycle progression in colon cancer cells. *Cancer Res* 2009;69:8157-65.

[127] Hatley ME, Patrick DM, Garcia MR, *et al*. Modulation of K-Ras-dependent lung tumorigenesis by MicroRNA-21. *Cancer Cell* 2010;18:282-93.

[128] Hennessey PT, Sanford T, Choudhary A, et al. Serum microRNA biomarkers for detection of non-small cell lung cancer. *PLoS One* 2012;7:e32307.

[129] Hammerman PS, Lawrence MS, and Voet D *et al*. The Cancer Genome Atlas Research Network. Comprehensive genomic characterization of squamous cell lung cancers. *Nature* 2012 Sep 9. doi: 10.1038/nature11404. [Epub ahead of print].

[130] Brambilla E, Lantuejoul S, Sturm N. Divergent differentiation in neuroendocrine lung tumors. *Semin Diagn Pathol* 2000;17:138–48.

[131] Wistuba II, Mao L, Gazdar AF. Smoking molecular damage in bronchial epithelium. *Oncogene* 2002;21:7298–306.

[132] Wistuba II, Gazdar AF. Characteristic genetic alterations in lung cancer. *Methods Mol Med* 2003;74:3-28.

[133] Jetten AM, Nervi C, Vollberg TM. Control of squamous differentiation in tracheobronchial and epidermal epithelial cells: role of retinoids. *J Natl Cancer Inst Monogr* 1992;320:93-100.

[134] Nettesheim P, Hammons AS. Induction of squamous cell carcinoma in the respiratory tract of mice. *J Natl Cancer Inst* 1971;47:697-701.

[135] Rehm S, Lijinsky W, Singh G, *et al*. Mouse bronchiolar cell carcinogenesis. Histologic characterization and expression of Clara cell antigen in lesions induced by N-nitroso-bis-(2-chloroethyl) ureas. *Am J Pathol* 1991;139:413-22.

[136] Wang Y, Zhang Z, Yan Y, *et al*. A chemically induced model for squamous cell carcinoma of the lung in mice: histopathology and strain susceptibility. *Cancer Res* 2004;64:1647-54.

[137] Dakir EL, Feigenbaum L, Linnoila RI. Constitutive expression of human keratin 14 gene in mouse lung induces premalignant lesions and squamous differentiation. *Carcinogenesis* 2008;29:2377-84.

[138] Ji H, Ramsey MR, Hayes DN, *et al*. LKB1 modulates lung cancer differentiation and metastasis. *Nature* 2007;448:807-10.

[139] Fisher GH, Wellen SL, Klimstra D, *et al*. Induction and apoptotic regression of lung adenocarcinomas by regulation of a K-Ras transgene in the presence and absence of tumor suppressor genes. *Genes Dev* 2001;15:3249-62.

[140] Politi K, Zakowski MF, Fan PD, *et al*. Lung adenocarcinomas induced in mice by mutant EGF receptors found in human lung cancers respond to a tyrosine kinase inhibitor or to down-regulation of the receptors. *Genes Dev* 2006;20:1496-510.

[141] Ji H, Li D, Chen L, *et al*. The impact of human EGFR kinase domain mutations on lung tumorigenesis and in vivo sensitivity to EGFR-targeted therapies. *Cancer Cell* 2006a;9:485-95.

[142] Ji H, Zhao X, Yuza Y, *et al*. Epidermal growth factor receptor variant III mutations in lung tumorigenesis and sensitivity to tyrosine kinase inhibitors. *Proc Natl Acad Sci USA* 2006b;103:7817-22.

[143] Engelman JA, Chen L, Tan X, *et al*. Effective use of PI3K and MEK inhibitors to treat mutant Kras G12D and PIK3CA H1047R murine lung cancers. *Nat Med* 2008;14:1351-6.

[144] Mahgoub N, Taylor BR, Gratiot M, *et al*. In vitro and in vivo effects of a farnesyltransferase inhibitor on Nf1-deficient hematopoietic cells. *Blood* 1999;94:2469-76.

[145] Omer CA, Chen Z, Diehl RE, *et al*. Mouse mammary tumor virus-Ki-rasB transgenic mice develop mammary carcinomas that can be growth-inhibited by a farnesyl:protein transferase inhibitor. *Cancer Res* 2000;60:2680-8.

[146] To MD, Wong CE, Karnezis AN, *et al*. Kras regulatory elements and exon 4A determine mutation specificity in lung cancer. *Nat Genet* 2008;40:1240-4.

[147] Contag CH, Jenkins D, Contag PR, *et al*. Use of reporter genes for optical measurements of neoplastic disease in vivo. *Neoplasia* 2000;2:41-52.

[148] Hadjantonakis AK, Dickinson ME, Fraser SE, *et al*. Technicolour transgenics: imaging tools for functional genomics in the mouse. *Nature Rev Genet* 2003;4:613-25.

[149] Jackson EL, Willis N, Mercer K, *et al*. Analysis of lung tumor initiation and progression using conditional expression of oncogenic K-ras. *Genes Dev* 2001;15:3243-8.

[150] Chen YQ, Zhou YQ, Fu LH, Wang D, Wang MH. Multiple pulmonary adenomas in the lung of transgenic mice overexpressing the RON receptor tyrosine kinase. Recepteur d'origine nantais. *Carcinogenesis* 2002;23:1811-9.

[151] O'Toole JM, Rabenau KE, Burns K, *et al*. Therapeutic implications of a human neutralizing antibody to the macrophage-stimulating protein receptor tyrosine kinase (RON), a c-MET family member. *Cancer Res* 2006;66:9162-70.

[152] Shames DS, Girard L, Gao B, *et al*. A genome-wide screen for promoter methylation in lung cancer identifies novel methylation markers for multiple malignancies. *PLoS Med* 2006; 3:e486.

[153] Shacter E, Weitzman SA. Chronic inflammation and cancer. *Oncology (Williston Park)*. 2002;16:217-26, 229; discussion 230-2.

[154] Vaid M, Floros J. Surfactant protein DNA methylation: a new entrant in the field of lung cancer diagnostics? *Oncol Rep* 2009;21:3-11.

[155] Korfhagen TR, Bruno MD, Ross GF, *et al*. Altered surfactant function and structure in SP-A gene targeted mice. *Proc Natl Acad Sci USA* 1996;93:9594-9.

[156] Botas C, Poulain F, Akiyama J, *et al*. Altered surfactant homeostasis and alveolar type II cell morphology in mice lacking surfactant protein D. *Proc Natl Acad Sci USA* 1998;95:11869–74.

Chapter 3

Relationship Between Toxicogenomic and Environment and Lung Cancer

M. Adonis, M. Chahuan, A. Zambrano, P. Avaria,
J. Díaz, R. Miranda, M. Campos, H. Benítez and L. Gil

Additional information is available at the end of the chapter

http://dx.doi.org/10.5772/55663

1. Introduction

Tobacco-smoke is associated with 75-90% of LC cases and ~50% occurs in developing countries (Parkin, et al. 2005; Parkin, et al. 1994). Several studies have demonstrated that organic and inorganic compounds are related with the development of cancer, including LC (Bradley and Golden 2006; De Palma, et al. 2008; Stavrides 2006). The association between cigarette smoking and various types of respiratory cancer has been demonstrated (U.S.EPA 2001) and many carcinogenic compounds present in cigarette smoke, such as polycyclic aromatic hydrocarbons (PAHs), have also been identified in airborne particles in different cities around the world (Adonis, et al. 1997; Gil, et al. 1995; Minoia, et al. 1997; Monarca, et al. 1998).

Cancer rates could further increase by 50% to 15 million new cases in the year 2020, according to the World Cancer Report (World Cancer Report, 2003). The report also reveals that cancer has emerged as a major public health problem in developing countries, matching its effect in industrialized nations. During 2008, more than 1.61 million of new LC cases and 1.31 million of deaths were reported worldwide (Ferlay et al, 2010), accounting for 13% of the total. More than half (55%), of the cases occurred in the developing countries. In South America the estimation for 2008, showed an incidence rate for men of 20.4 /100,000 inhabitant and a mortality rate of 18.8 /100,000 inhabitant (WHO, 2008). For the same period, the women showed a rates/100,000 inhabitant of 8.4 for incidence and 7.4 for mortality.

PAHs are metabolized to reactive DNA binding diols epoxides by phase I enzymes as cytochrome P4501A1 (CYP1A1) and detoxified by phase II enzymes as GSTs, before reaching their target. Adonis et al (2005), have proposed that the contribution of individual variations in metabolic activities of each or both phases, in regulating the clearance of DNA toxic metabolites, are at least partially related to the individual host susceptibility to PAHs. Several polymorphisms have been described in CYP1A1, however, 3′noncoding region (Msp1, CYP1A1*2A) has been the most studied (Gil et al, 1992; Adonis et al. 1997, Quiñones et al, 2001; Adonis et al, 2005a, 2005b, Ji et al, 2012).

Additionally, the association between inorganic Arsenic (iAs) and skin, bladder, and lung carcinogenesis has been well-established. It is estimated than 220 million in 105 countries are exposed worldwide to iAs (Murcott, 2012). In the Northern Chilean region of Antofagasta, the population (close to 500,000 inhabitants) have been chronically exposed to As concentrations as high as 870 $\mu g\ l^{-1}$ from 1958 through 1970, with some towns still registering concentrations of 600 $\mu g\ l^{-1}$ by the year 2000 (Smith et al, 1998). This has occurred despite international guidelines placing the maximum tolerable arsenic exposure at 10 $\mu g\ l^{-1}$ (IARC, 2004).

As occurs naturally in soil, water and air, the main sources of environmental As exposure in Chile are copper smelters and drinking water (Queirolo et al., 2000; De Gregori et al, 2003). Chile, with a population close to 17.1 million (http://data.worldbank.org/country/chile) and a total life expectancy at birth of 78 years, shows a high rate of lung cancer (LC), especially in the North of Chile. During 2007, Chile showed more than 2,500 LC cases and 1,900 deaths. Between 1990 and 2008 the LC national mortality rate/100.000 inhabitants for both gender increased since 10.8 to 14.6; while for the period 2003–2007, the Antofagasta region (Northern Chile) showed a rate mortality of 30.8/100.000, the second rate mortality higher after skin cancer (Vallebuona, 2011). To stratify by gender, the Antofagasta region for the same period showed for men the highest LC rate mortality/100.000 (53.1), higher than prostate (38.9), and skin (50.4).

The mechanism by which As causes cancer is still no clear and has been speculated that its carcinogenicity potency in humans might be modulate by concurrent exposure to other agents that modify the risk of cancer to As, as environmental pollution containing high levels of carcinogen compounds (Adonis et al, 2005) and or smoking (Thomas et al, 2001), as well as both genetic and epigenetic processes (Salnikow and Zhitkovich, 2008). As is metabolized through a series of reductions of pentavalents to trivalent species, followed by oxidative methylations to yield pentavalent methylated species. It is well recognized that inorganic As is methylated to monomethyl As acid (MMA) and dimethyl As acid (DMA) with a methyl group from S-adenosylmethionine. As reduction of As to the trivalent form is a prerequisite for oxidative methylation, pentavalent arsenicals are reduced by endogenous thiols such as glutathione (GSH) or by As^{V} reductases (Kala el al., 2000; Radabaugh & Aposhian, 2000, Zakharyan et al., 2001; Radabaugh et al., 2002). Liver is the main site of methylation, but methylation activity is present in all tissues (Vahter, 2002). Arsenic3 methyltransferase (As3MT) is the key enzyme in the biotransformation of iAs. As3MT catalyzes the transfer of a methyl group from S-adenosyl-methionine to trivalent arsenicals resulting in the production of Monometil As(MAs) and dimethylated arsenicals *3 (DMAs). MAs is a susceptibility factor of iAs induced toxicity, before to be excreted in the urine.

As was mentioned before, the high incidence of lung cancer (LC) has been associated with cigarette smoking, however genetic diversity and environmental pollution must also be considered as risk factors, especially in those cities highly exposed to environmental carcinogens. Although, there are many advances in the disease control, very little is known about changes in detection of pre neoplastic, pre invasive lesions or in the initial steps in LC development. LC has been described as one of the most aggressive diseases with multiples genomic changes or alterations in specific fragments of the DNA, some of them including genes associated with the cell system preservation within normal parameters. Some of the changes might promote a transformation from a normal cell into a tumour cell in a multistage process.

The genomic age, the new images technologies and informatics, probably will demand in a short time from the government, health professionals (clinic and basic), public and private institutions, etc., new actions to improve the public health.

Cancer diagnosis can be done in different stages of the disease. The cancer diagnosis has as main objectives to know the localization (place) and also to identify the stage (stage) and the histological characterization (kind). The knowledge of the place, stage and kind will help to define the treatment and will determine the survival and the clinic success. For LC the current technologies are arriving late, indeed more than 85% of the LC patients died after the diagnosis (McWilliams et al, 2009; Nakamura et al., 2001; Kennedy et al., 2007; Woolner et al., 1984). The main reason of the high mortality is related with the small fraction of the patients detected in early stages. This is mainly related with absence of symptoms in an early stage.

Obviously, the early diagnosis will load in the clinic success in term of treatment and survival. The use of new technologies as complementary tools might chance or improve the early detection and the treatment success. The use of the advanced technologies might reduce the mortality, thus it is possible not only detect early stages but also to have early treatment.

Early detection has a direct relationship with the population screening, in order to identify risk population, healthy population and or asymptomatic population, especially for LC asymptomatic in the early stages. Smoking habit is probably the main risk factor for LC, however additional factors might contribute to the risk of LC. Among the LC risk factors is valid to mention environmental pollution, occupational exposure, life style and genetic factors. That mean, that among the population is possible to find people with a high risk of LC, which would be the main candidates to a screening programme to detect pre neoplastic lesions or early stages.

Within some of the news or advances technologies can be mentioned, Quantitative Automatic Cytology (QAC), Autofluorescence-reflectance bronchoscopy (AFB) and the tumor biomarker DR70, used in a pilot study for early detection of LC, in a high risk population. These technologies have been studied in Chile in a LC risk population, exposed to high levels of air pollutants (Santiago) and on the other hand to high historical exposure to As in drinking water (Antofagasta). Part of these results, were presented in an oral presentation, titled "Pilot Study for Lung Cancer and Pre neoplastic Lesions", in the XXX1 Word Congress of Internal Medicine (WCIM, 2012), where the work got the Award for the First Best Research Work. This is a report of an ongoing prospective bimodality cancer surveillance study for high risk LC volunteers. This study has been done in 364 people, exposed naturally to environmental pollution and where the biomarkers, QAC and DR70 (Onko Sure), were used as tools in the detection of preneoplastic lesions (PNL) and neoplastic lesions (NL). The study has also included Autofluorescent Bronchoscopy (AFB) as an additional technique, to detect pre neoplastic or pre invasive lesions in the voluntaries with high likehood of malignance for LC, according to AQC and DR70.

2. Materials and methods

The people that were interested and met the criteria for the inclusion factors were enrolled as voluntaries (Figure 1).

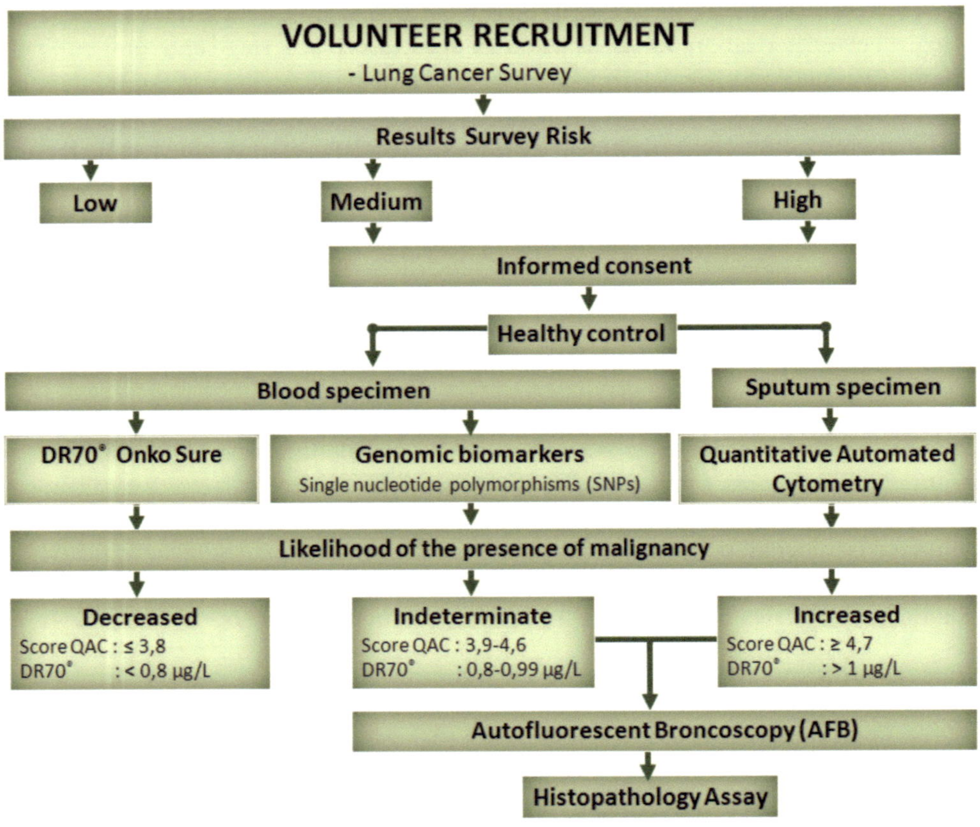

Figure 1. Diagram of the enrolling process for recruiting the voluntaries for LC prevention.

The high risk subjects for LC were recruited via advertisement in newspaper, radio and internet (University of Chile web) and were included in this study from two regions of Chile, Metropolitan (Santiago city) and Antofagasta. Enrolment was based on a LC Risk Survey (Witteman et al., 2011) by Washington University School of Medicine, which was modified by our group. Subjects were eligible for enrolment procedure if they met the following criteria's: male/female aged 40 years or older; family history of LC, non-smokers and ever smokers exposed naturally to environmental air pollution (Metropolitan region) or to arsenic in drinking water (Antofagasta region) for at least 10 years.

In addition, we enrolled subjects who were suspected of having lung cancer (N=12) based on their clinical symptoms, with the final diagnosis completed in the study. These patients did not have previous tests performed on them such as cytology or CT and did not have any treatment. However, only 12 of them were in agreement to undergo to the AFB, while all of them underwent a CT to rule out or confirm the LC.

The voluntaries were classified according to their risk score, which allowed for classification of the subjects in three risk categories: low, medium and high. Subjects with medium or high risk were invited to participate in the study. The LC risk predictor was applied to 508 volunteer participants, obtaining 364 subjects with medium to high-risk for LC. Of those, 224 were from Santiago and 140 were from the Antofagasta's region.

Sputum generation was induced by inhalation of 3% saline solution, after administration of two puffs of salbutamol. Patients were instructed to cough and expectorate before their Specimens were collected in 50 mL centrifuge tubes, followed by adding enough SedFix solution. Each tube was mixed with DTT solution and was shaken at 1800 rpm overnight. After centrifugation, a cell pellet was obtained; re suspended in an ethanol solution and was placed on slides. The cell DNA was stained with Feulgen thionin and was analysed by an automated cytometry-based scoring system, as described by Kemp et al. (Kemp et al, 2007).

Furthermore, blood samples were taken in serum separator tubes in the morning before ingestion of any meal. The tubes were left at room temperature for 30 minutes. The serum was separated from the cells by centrifugation at 3,500 rpm for 10 min. Each serum specimen was diluted 1:200 with the diluent buffer and was tested along with the calibrators according to AMDL Diagnostics Onko Sure protocol (Radient Pharmaceuticals) as described in Adonis et al. (2005) and Hatton et al. (2006).

Participants with positive DR70 test (threshold>1.0), or an AQC score ≥4.6 were invited to have an AFB, using the Onco-LIFE device (Novadaq Inc., Richmond, Canada), under local anaesthesia. The airways were examined by, White Light Broncoscopy (WLB) and Auto Fluorescence Broncoscopy (AFB) and the visual findings were classified as normal, abnormal or suspicious, as described by Lam et al. (1998). Endobronchial mucosal biopsies were taken from all areas that were suspicious under WLB or AFB. In addition, surveillance biopsies were taken from epithelium with normal appearance in all subjects. An average of 2-3 biopsies was taken from each of the participants.

Categorical variables were analysed by Fisher's exact test. Sensitivity, specificity, likelihood ratio (LR), Predictive Positive Value (PPV) and Predictive Negative Value (PNV) were calculated with 95% CI. Statistical significance was accepted at $p<0.05$. The sensitivity and specificity were assessed for each test and was used in analysis as a single test; two-test parallel combination and two-test series combination (Sullivan and Thomson, 2000, Kruskal, 1998).

3. Results

As show the Figure 2, 27.4% of subjects display an AQC with an increased likelihood of malignancy (score equal or higher than 4.6) and 26.1% showed undetermined likelihood of malignancy (score between 3.9 and < 4.6). Among samples with increased AQC (27.4 %), 15.75% and 11.68% were negative and positive (≥ 1 µg/mL) for DR70, respectively. Samples with undetermined AQC showed 22.01% and 4.07% of negative and positive DR70 values, respectively. Among 46.5% of samples that showed decreased likelihood of malignancy, 42.11% were negative and 4.34% were positive for DR70. In the latter group, additional clinical tests confirmed several cancers including colon, breast and one case of prostate cancer, currently under study.

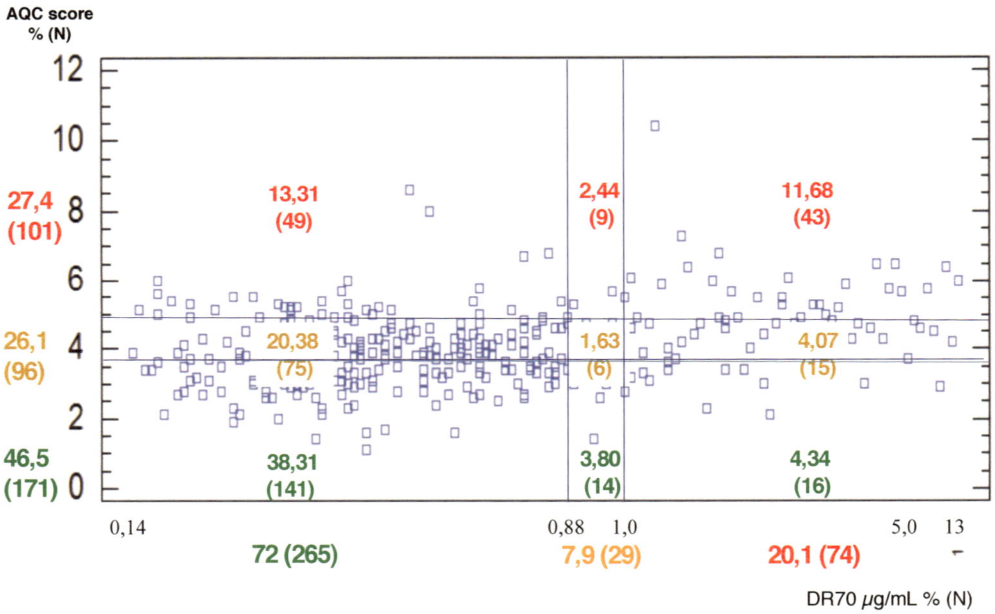

Figure 2. AQC and DR70 correlation and percentage (N) for each LC risk interval. Likehood LC risk: AQC: ≥ 4.6, increased; ≥ 3.9 ≤ 4.6 undetermined; ≤ 3.9 decreased DR70: ≥ 1.0, increased; ≤ 1.0 decreased

The data shows that DR70 itself might contribute to confirm tumour diagnosis and to identify patients with advanced LC, with high sensitivity (Table 3). However, the test would be better identifying negative LC cases with a high specificity and Negative Predictive Value (NPV). AQC for itself resulted with high sensitivity and specificity for LC with higher NPV than Negative Predictive Value (PPV), confirming especially negative tests, with high precision. Related to PNL, both biomarkers might be used as complementary tools to confirm negativity for PNL, showing a higher specificity (98.6%) than both test for itself, keeping a high NPV (97.2%).

On the other hand, AFB identified PNL (metaplasia and dysplasia) better than the White Light Bronchoscopy (WLB) by itself. As show the Figure 3, AFB detected a zone with a score of 0.67, suspicious of malignance and normal according to WLB. The Histopathology assay informed for the biopsy taking in this zone, increasing in the coarse epithelial and desmosomes and cellular flatting and maturation in the upper layer; in comparison to a normal epithelium (Figure 3B), without cytology atypias; classifying the biopsy as a Squamous metaplasia (Figure 3A).

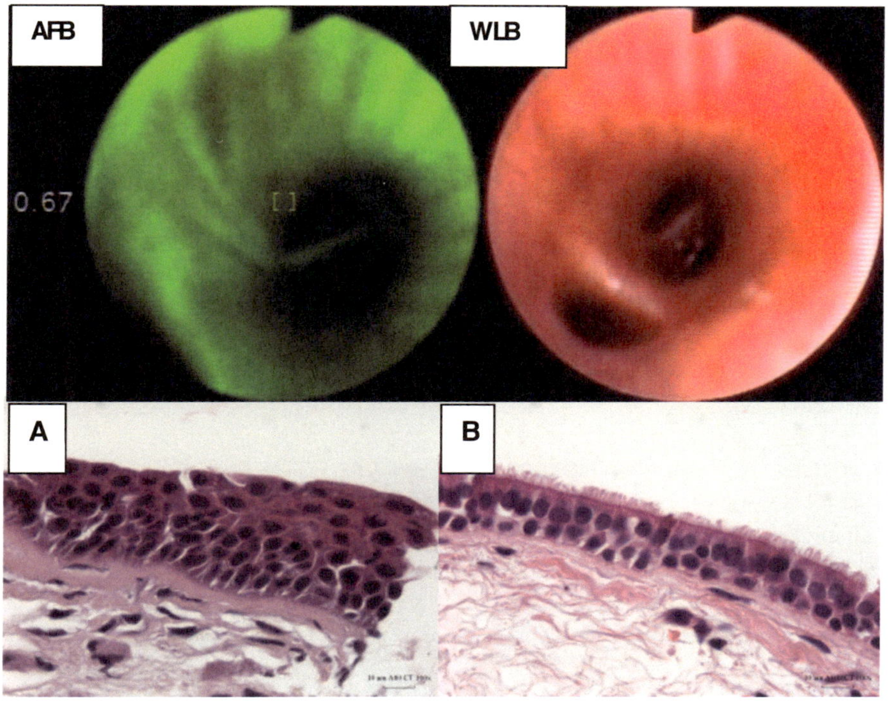

Figure 3. AFB and WLB and Histopathology assay for a Squamous Metaplasia Volunteer A80. Squamous Metaplasia (B) Volunteer A109. Normal Epithelium Stain HE 100x. CeteCáncer. INNOVA CORFO. Thesis Avaria P. MSc, Faculty of Medicine, University of Chile, 2012

The Figure 4 shows an AFB with a score of 0.83 and suspicious of malignance. The Histopathology assay informed a considerable cellular increasing in the 2/3 lower, pleomorphism, nuclear heterogeneity, chromatin density increased without mitosis, classifying the biopsy as mild dysplasia (Figure 4A).

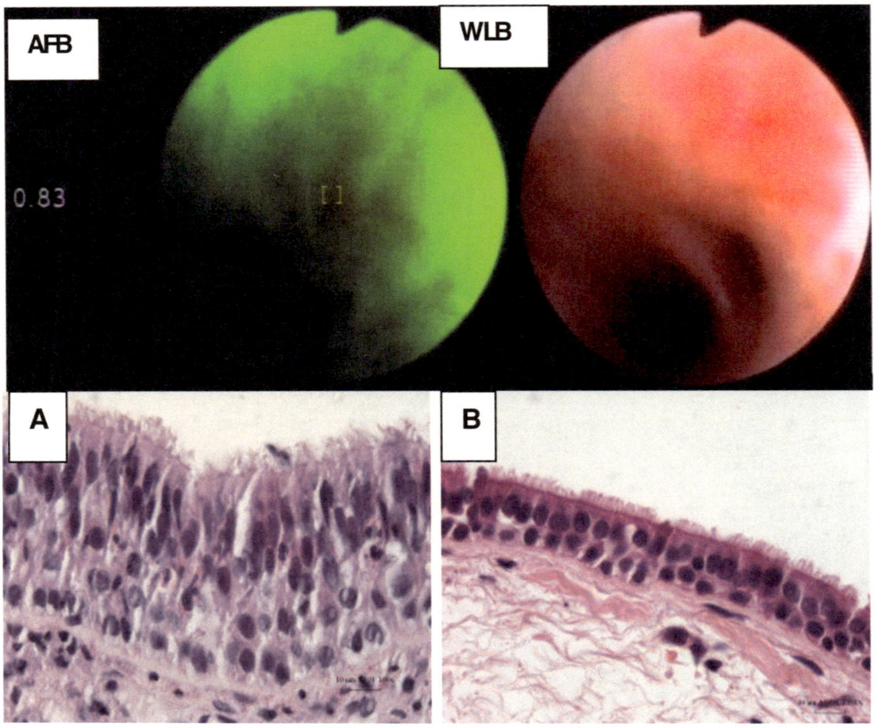

Figure 4. AFB and WLB and Histopathology assay for a Mild Dysplasia Volunteer A101. Mild Dysplasia (B) Volunteer A109. Normal Epithelium Stain HE 100x. CeteCáncer. INNOVA CORFO. Thesis Avaria P. MSc, Faculty of Medicine, University of Chile, 2012

Fifty percent of the samples, classified as suspicious (12%) by AFB, were confirmed as metaplasia (33%) or dysplasia (17%) by histopathology. The rest of the samples classified by AFB as suspicious were classified by the histopathology as inflammation (25%) and hyperplasia (25%). Non one was related with a normal histopathology sample (Figure 5).

Biomarkers	Sensitivity % (IC 95%)		Specificity % (IC95%)	
	LC	PNL	LC	PNL
DR70	95.8 (784,9- 99,0)	27.3 (6.0 -61.0)	91.9 (88.1-94.8)	91.9 (88.1-94.3)
AQC	64.0 (42.5- 82.0)	90.9 (58.7- 99.8)	89.4 (85.2-92.7)	89.4 (85.2-92.7)

Table 1. Sensitivity and Specificity for DR70 and AQC, for LC and PNL

The data shows that DR70 itself might contribute to confirm tumour diagnosis and to identify patients with advanced LC, with high sensitivity (95.8%) and specificity (91.9%) (Table 1). AQC

http://dx.doi.org/10.5772/55663

for itself resulted with high sensitivity and specificity for LC, but showed a higher sensitivity and specificity than DR70 for PNL, 90.9% and 89.4%, respectively. Additionally, both biomarkers might be used as complementary tools to confirm negativity for LC and or PNL. In conclusion, as a pre screener for LC, both biomarkers test might be employed with at high specificity/high sensitivity as complementary tools to detect LC. For PNL, both tests would be better confirming negativity than subjecting presence of PNL.

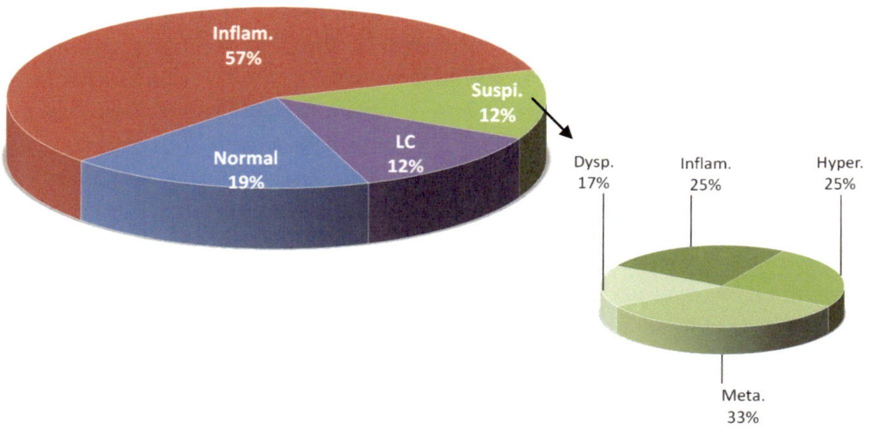

Figure 5. Relationship between Autofluorescence Broncoscopy (AFB) and Histopathology Assay (HA)

4. Discussion

This is the first study in Latin America to complement image techniques with cellular and molecular biomarkers, to detect LC and PNL. These results provide scientific and clinical information for Chilean health authorities to include early detection of LC in the AUGE government programme, that provide additional health services for patients.

Our results presented here clearly demonstrate the reliability of both biomarkers to select good candidates for detect LC or pre neoplasic lesions (PNL). These results suggest that both AQC and DR70 might provide transcendentally information not only to confirm or suggest diagnostic for LC, but also to surveillance screening of LC after treatment. It is as important to confirm diagnostic as predict a patient's response to certain cancer therapies or determine whether cancer has returned.

These results obtained via biomarkers in blood and sputum were quite promising in elucidating risk to LC, especially when the biomarkers studied are non invasive and inexpensive assays and could be an effective methods also to monitor the biological effects of environmental and occupational carcinogens.

Additionally, we presented evidences that showed that AFB is more sensitive than WLB to detect early lesions, thereby allowing their localisation for biopsy or interventional procedures. Then the association of WLB and AFB would increase the sensitivity to detect PNL.

Is well known that resolution of CT scan and other images technologies improves each year, allowing to detect more nodules, but not necessarily LC in early stages. Additionally, is well known the high frequency of lung nodules with undetermined significance and that LC often causes no symptoms until it is spread outside the lung. From this point of view, non invasive biomarkers and AFB might contribute as a first step in detecting pre- neoplastic a pre- invasive lesions. Screening in people with high LC risk including those with smoking habit and or nodules non necessary cancerous, might means a higher survival and improve the life quality. The screening in people with high risk of LC might be a good preventive way to improve the survival to 5 years, especially when different studies have shown an important association between genetic host characteristics and exposure to environmental carcinogens.

Genetic differences in metabolic activation and detoxification of environmental carcinogen, like PAHs and or As, may partially explain host susceptibility to chemically induced cancers (Daly et al., 1994; London et al, 2000, Kang et al, 2012).

Adonis et al (2005) showed the association of combined genotypes of cytochrome CYP1A1 (Msp1) and glutathione-S-transferase GSTM1 and lung cancer risk, for a population historically exposed to As in the Antofagasta region. This study showed in the healthy group, a CYP1A1 *2A allele frequency for MspI of 0.41, whereas for lung cancer group 0.46. No statically significant difference was observed between the healthy group and lung cancer group (p = 0.437, CI =–0.224 to 0.124). However, the CYP1A1 *2A genotype was associated with an increased relative lung cancer risk O.R. = 2.08 (95% CI = 1.04–4.03, p = 0.04). In addition, 35% of healthy group and 39% of the lung cancer group were homozygote for the null variant allele of GSTM1. For men the CYP1A1 *2A genotype was associated with a highly significant estimated relative lung cancer risk O.R. = 2.60 (95% CI = 1.07–5.94, p = 0.0334). The relative lung cancer risk for the total sample with the CYP1A1 *2A/null GSTM1 genotype was 2.51 (O.R. = 2.51, CI = 1.07–5.40, p = 0.0322), which one increased when the sample was stratified by smoking habit (O.R. = 2.98, CI = 1.10–7.10, p = 0.0497) (Adonis et al, 2005).

These results suggest that patients with previous history of iAs exposure as the Antofagasta population, and with smoking habit might be have an additional factor related to genetic susceptibility to lung cancer. The cancer mortality rate in region II for iAs- associated cancers, as lung cancer, at least might be partly related to differences in As biotransformation. Individuals with the CYP1A1*2A and/or the combined CYP1A1*2A and GSTM1 null genotype might have a greater capacity to metabolically active PAHs and lower capacity to conjugate with glutathione and clearance of As, which may result in a higher risk of lung cancer or respiratory tract illness.

One of the main conclusion is there is an interaction between CYP1A1 polymorphism, GSTM1 null genotype and LC risk, especially in people exposed to carcinogenic compounds like to As and PAHs. In conclusion, genetic biomarkers such as CYP1A1 and GSTM1 polymorphisms in addition to other genetic biomarkers and other biomarkers like to QAC and DR70 and clinical tools might provide relevant information to identify individuals at high risk to lung cancer as prevention and protection actions of public health.

Acknowledgements

This work was supported by Grants from INNOVA-CORFO Chile (07CN13PBT-48 and 11IDL2-10634, 2012). We also thank all the volunteers that accepted to participate in this project and to the permanent support of the Canada Embassy in Chile. The authors also thank Dr. Stephen Lam for his invaluable support, advise and helpful discussions. This work has been carried out with ethical committee approval of the Faculty of Medicine of University of Chile.

Author details

M. Adonis[1], M. Chahuan[2], A. Zambrano[3], P. Avaria[1], J. Díaz[1], R. Miranda[4], M. Campos[2], H. Benítez[3] and L. Gil[1]

1 CeTeCáncer, Faculty of Medicine, University of Chile, Chile

2 San Borja Arriaran Hospital, Chile

3 Antofagasta Regional Hospital, Chile

4 Barros Lucos Trudeau Hospital, Chile

References

[1] Adonis, M, Quinones, L, Gil, L, & Gibson, G. (1997). Hepatic enzyme induction and mutagenicity of airborne particulate matter from Santiago, Chile in the nourished and malnourished rat. Xenobiotica: , 27(5), 527-36.

[2] Adonis, M, Martínez, V, Marín, P, Berrios, D, & Gil, L. (2005). Smoking habit and genetic factors associated with lung cancer in a population highly exposed to arsenic. Toxicol Lett: , 159(1), 32-7.

[3] Bradley, T. P, & Golden, A. L. Tobacco and carcinogens in the workplace. Clin Occup Environ Med. (2006). , 5(1), 117-37.

[4] Daly, A. K, Cholerton, S, Armstrong, M, & Idle, J. R. (1994). Genotyping for polymorphisms in xenobiotic metabolism as a predictor of disease susceptibility. Environ Health Perspect.; 102 Suppl , 9, 55-61.

[5] De Palma, G, Goldoni, M, Catalani, S, Carbognani, P, Poli, D, Mozzoni, P, Acampa, O, Internullo, E, Rusca, M, & Apostoli, P. Metallic elements in pulmonary biopsies from lung cancer and control subjects. Acta Biomed. (2008). Suppl , 1, 43-51.

[6] Ferlay, J, Shin, H. R, Bray, F, Forman, D, Mathers, C, Parkin, D. M, & Globocan, v. Cancer Incidence and Mortality Worldwide: IARC CancerBase Internet] Lyon, France: International Agency for Research on Cancer, 2010. Available from: http://globocan.iarc.fr.Accessed May 2011.(10)

[7] Gil, L, Adonis, M, Cáceres, D, & Moreno, G. (1995). Impact of outdoor pollution on indoor air quality. The case of downtown Santiago (Chile).Rev Med Chile: , 123(4), 411-25.

[8] Hatton, M. W, Southward, S. M, Ross, B. L, Clarke, B. J, Singh, G, & Richardson, M. (2006). Relationships among tumor burden, tumor size, and the changing concentrations of fibrin degradation products and fibrinolytic factors in the pleural effusions of rabbits with VX2 lung tumors. J Lab Clin Med.;, 147(1), 27-35.

[9] Kang, J, Koo, S, Kwon, K, & Park, J. (2010). Frequent silence of chromosome 9p, homozygous dock8, dmrt1 and dmrt3 deletion at 9in squamous cell carcinoma of the lung. International Journal of Oncology 37: 327-335, 2010, 24.

[10] Kemp, R. A, Reinders, D. M, & Turic, B. (2007). Detection of Lung Cancer by Automated Sputum Cytometry. Journal of Thoracic Oncology: 2 (11), 993-1000.

[11] Kennedy, T. C, Mcwilliams, A, Edell, E, et al. American College of Chest Physicians. Bronchial intraepithelial neoplasia/early central airways lung cancer: ACCP evidence-based clinical practice guidelines (2nd edition). Chest (2007). Suppl. 3 221S-233S.

[12] Kruskal, W. H. (1980). The significance of Fisher: A review of R. A. Fisher. The Life of a Scientist, by Joan Fisher Box. Journal of the American Statistical Association, , 75, 1019-1030.

[13] Lam, S, Kennedy, T, & Unger, M. (1998). Localization of bronchial intraepithelial neoplastic lesions by fluorescence bronchoscopy. Chest: , 113, 696-702.

[14] London, S. J, Smart, J, & Daly, A. K. (2000). Lung cancer risk in relation to genetic polymorphisms of microsomal epoxide hydrolase among African-Americans and Caucasians in Los Angeles County. Lung Cancer, , 28(2), 147-55.

[15] Mcwilliams, A, Lam, B, & Sutedja, T. Early proximal lung cancer diagnosis and treatment. Eur Respir J. (2009). Mar;, 33(3), 656-65.

[16] Minoia, C, Magnaghi, S, Micoli, G, Fiorentino, M. L, Turci, R, Angeleri, S, & Berri, A. (1997). Determination of environmental reference concentration of six PAHs in urban areas (Pavia, Italy). Sci Total Environ: , 198(1), 33-41.

[17] Monarca, S, Zanardini, A, Feretti, D, Falistocco, E, Antonelli, P, Resola, S, Moretti, M, Villarini, M, & Nardi, G. Mutagenicity and clastogenicity of gas stove emissions in bacterial and plant tests. Environ Mol Mutagen: , 31(4), 402-8.

[18] Murcott, S. Arsenic contamination in the word. (2012). 978-1-78040-038-9, 368.

[19] Nakamura, H, Kawasaki, N, Hagiwara, M, et al. Early hilar lung cancer- risk for multiple lung cancers and clinical outcome. Lung Cancer (2001). , 33, 51-57.

[20] Parkin, D. M, Bray, F, Ferlay, J, & Pisani, P. (2005). Global cancer statistics, 2002. CA Cancer J Clin , 55(2), 74-108.

[21] Parkin, D. M, Pisani, P, Lopez, A. D, & Masuyer, E. (1994). At least one in seven cases of cancer is caused by smoking. Global estimates for 1985. Int J Cancer , 59(4), 494-504.

[22] Stavrides, J. C. Lung carcinogenesis: pivotal role of metals in tobacco smoke. Free Radic Biol Med. (2006). , 41(7), 1017-30.

[23] Sullivan, M, & Thomson, M. (2000). Combining diagnostic test results to increase accuracy. Biostatistics. 1, 2: 123-140.

[24] US- EPA. Arsenic in drinking water rule (66 FR 6976 / January 22, 2001) http://water.epa.gov/lawsregs/rulesregs/sdwa/arsenic/index.cfm. EPA (U.S. Environmental Protection Agency). 2001. National Primary Drinking Water Regulations. Arsenic and Clarifications to Compilance and New Source Contaminants Monitoring. Final rule. Delay of effective date. Federal Registry. p 16134-16135.

[25] Vallebuona(2011). EPIDEMIOLOGICA DE CANCER Viña del Mar, Septiembre 2011. Ministerio de Salud Gobierno de Chile.

[26] World Health Organization. WHO report on the Global Tobacco Epidemic, (2008). the MPOWER package 2008, Geneva: World Health Organisation. http://data.worldbank.org/country/chile

[27] Witteman, H, Zikmund-fisher, B, Waters, E, Gavaruzzi, T, & Fagerlin, A. (2011). Risk estimates from an online risk calculator are more believable and recalled better when expressed as integres. Cancer Prevention Faculty Publications Cancer Prevention. Washington University School of Medicine. Journal of Medical Internet Research.; 13(3): 54.

[28] Woolner, L, Fontana, R, Cortese, D, et al. Roentgenographically occult lung cancer; pathologic findings and frequency of multicentricity during a 10-year period. Mayo Clin Proc (1984). , 59, 453-466.

Section 2

Inflammation and the Lung

Chapter 4

Acute Exacerbations of Chronic Obstructive Pulmonary Disease

S. Uzun, R.S. Djamin, H.C. Hoogsteden,
J.G.J.V. Aerts and M.M. van der Eerden

Additional information is available at the end of the chapter

http://dx.doi.org/10.5772/54867

1. Introduction

Chronic obstructive pulmonary disease (COPD) is a disease which is characterized by airway inflammation and progressive airflow limitation with poor reversibility. Patients with COPD can experience periods of acute deterioration, which are called exacerbations. There are different definitions for an acute exacerbation of COPD (AECOPD). A symptom reported AECOPD is defined solely based on a patient's symptoms [1]. This is regardless of whether the patient seeks medical attention or receives treatment for the exacerbation. An event defined AECOPD requires a therapeutic intervention such as a change in COPD medications or a change in healthcare utilization [1]. Generally accepted is the definition as in the guidelines of the World Health Organization, US National Heart Lung and Blood Institute and Global Initiative for Chronic Obstructive Lung Disease (GOLD), which define an exacerbation as "an event in the natural course of the disease characterized by a change in the patient's baseline dyspnoea, cough, and/or sputum that is beyond normal day-to-day variations, is acute in onset and may warrant a change in regular medication in a patient with COPD" [2]. Frequent exacerbations can result in a decreased health related quality of life [3], a decline in lung function [4], an increased risk of hospitalization [5] and an increase in mortality [6].

COPD and acute exacerbations of COPD (AECOPD) impose a burden on health care and society. It is estimated that COPD is the 4th leading cause of death worldwide and will be the 3rd leading cause of death in 2030 [7]. Along with increasing mortality rates, the loss in disability-adjusted life years (DALYs) also rises. By 2030 COPD will be the 5th leading cause of loss in DALYs globally, where it was only number 13 in 2004. Increasing health care costs will be the consequence of this trend. In the European Union COPD accounts for just over 3% of the total health care budget. In the USA, the direct and indirect costs for COPD are almost 50 billion USD. The majority of these costs are attributed to exacerbations [8]. The importance of exacerbations is reflected in the latest update of the GOLD report, in which the number of exacerbations in the preceding year is incorporated in the new classification of a patient with COPD [8]. In order to try to reduce the mortality, loss in DALYs and related costs and to lower the burden on society and health care, it is a goal to prevent and treat COPD and exacerbations of COPD. This chapter will give a concise overview of the background of AECOPD and the available tools for its treatment and prevention.

2. Epidemiology

The prevalence of COPD varies greatly per country and also within countries [9]. This heterogeneity can be contributed to not only differences in diagnostic methods and classification but also to smoking habits, population age, in- and outdoor air pollution, occupational exposure, prevalence of pulmonary tuberculosis, chronic asthma and socioeconomic status [10]. Prevalences of COPD have been reported varying from 0,2-37% [11, 12]. The prevalence of AECOPD is very difficult to determine since there is no generally agreed definition for an AECOPD (see above). Studies show that only 32-50% of symptom defined AECOPD are reported by patients to health care professionals [13, 14]. Although there is no reliable estimate of the prevalence of AECOPD, much is known about the occurrence of exacerbations. Research shows that exacerbations are more frequent in the winter season [15] and may occur clustered in time [16]. Exacerbations are also more frequent and severe as COPD severity increases [17]. Besides COPD severity, the history of exacerbations is also a good predictor of future exacerbations [17]. Furthermore, there is a strong correlation with symptoms of depression and recurrent exacerbations [18, 19].

3. Pathophysiology of COPD and AECOPD

COPD is the result of a chronic inflammation in the airways. The inflammation is initiated by chronic exposure to exogenic toxins (e.g. cigarette smoke) which is causing damage to the airway epithelium and is activating the innate immune system giving a rapid, nonspecific response [20, 21]. Of the innate immune response the neutrophillic inflammation is most prominent in COPD. The cells of the innate immune system activate the adaptive immune system, of which CD8+-cells, CD4+ $T_{helper}1$ cells and B-cells have an important role in COPD. This activation of the adaptive immune response is the beginning of a cascade which causes extensive chronic inflammation, oxidative stress and remodeling, resulting in destruction of alveolar space and deposition of connective tissue in the subepithelium and adventitium of the airway wall [22]. The degree of chronic inflammation in COPD correlates with the severity of airflow limitation. This is supported by a correlation which is seen between the severity of obstruction and presence of CD8+-cells and B-cells in the small conducting airways [22] and the presence of neutrophils in sputum [23]. Also, bacterial colonization is more frequently observed in patients with severe to very severe COPD, suggesting that bacterial colonization induces inflammation and contributes to the progression of COPD [24, 25]. The existence of the chronic inflammation and oxidative stress is supported by the presence of oxidants and numerous pro-inflammatory cytokines in the airways and serum. Compared to healthy controls, sputum specimens of patients with stable COPD and AECOPD show increased numbers of neutrophils and increased levels of pro-inflammatory cytokines like interleukin-6 (IL-6) and interleukin-8 (IL-8) [21, 23, 26-29]. During an AECOPD neutrophils, IL-6 and IL-8 are also increased in serum [27, 30, 31]. Interleukin-6 is a cytokine released during initial immune response by different cell types of the native immune system, like macrophages. It induces hepatic acute phase response during inflammation [32] which in turn increases production of C-reactive protein (CRP). Interleukin-6 is also a growth factor for T- and B-cells [33]. Interleuking-8 is released by a variety of cell types involved in inflammation, like endothelial cells, fibroblasts and monocytes [34]. It is a potent neutrophil chemotactic and activating factor [34]. The presence of the increased inflammation in serum both during stable state and AECOPD may be explained by the "overspill theory", in which the local inflammatory processes in the lung "spill over" to the systemic circulation [35]. It is therefore thought that disease activity of COPD can be measured in serum by biomarkers. Exhaled breath condensate (EBC) components are thought to reflect the physiological state of lining fluid of the airways. It's a non-invasive mean of obtaining information on oxidative stress and inflammation in the airways. Hydrogen peroxide (H_2O_2, a precursor of potent oxidants OH and HOCl) and 8-isoprostane (formed by the free radical peroxidation of arachidonic acid) are EBC oxidative stress biomarkers proven to be elevated in patients with COPD during stable state and during exacerbations [31, 36-38]. Heme-oxygenase-1 (HO-1) is an inducible catalyzer of the degradation of heme to biliverdin which is thought to provide protection from oxidative stress. It is decreased in ex-smokers with COPD compared to control subjects [39] but increased during severe exacerbations [29], in healthy smokers and current smokers with COPD [40].

4. Aetiology of AECOPD

4.1. Microbiology

There is a great variety in reported infectious causes of COPD exacerbations. It is of importance to determine, both for bacteria and viruses, whether the presence of the microbe is actually the cause of the exacerbation. Estimated is that about 50-78% of acute exacerbations of COPD are caused by respiratory infections [24, 27, 41, 42], in which the clinical presentation range from pneumonia to coryzal symptoms with dyspnea. Patients with AECOPD of proven infectious aetiology have a longer hospital stay and a greater decrease in FEV_1 than patients with non-infective exacerbations [27].

4.2. Viral causes

In the past viruses have been an underestimated cause of AECOPD and the causative role of viruses in AECOPD is still not fully established. The observation that as well viral infections and exacerbations are seasonal does suggest that viruses have a role in AECOPD [15, 43].

Recently researchers deliberately exposed patients with COPD and healthy smokers to rhinoviruses and observed that this virus was able to cause an exacerbation in patients with COPD [44]. Detection of viruses by culture and by serology, where a second serum sample is also required, is less sensitive and more time consuming than PCR techniques, where only 1 sample is required. Because of the advanced PCR techniques in detecting viruses, the percentage of exacerbations they account for can also be overestimated. The presence of viral DNA or RNA does not implicate that the virus is the cause of an exacerbation as several studies reported patients with stable COPD to carry viruses with percentages varying from 12-19% [45, 46]. In exacerbations several studies have reported that viruses were detected in 20-56% of cases [24, 27, 41, 42, 46, 47]. In these studies rhinovirus, influenza virus and respiratory syncytial virus and were the most common isolated viruses. A more extensive overview can be found in table 1.

COPD exacerbations: divided by cause	
Bacteria	
	Streptococcus pneumoniae
	Haemophilus influenzae
	Moraxella catarrhalis
	Haemophilus parainfluenzae
	Pseudomonas aeruginosa
	Staphylococcus aureus
Viruses	
	Human rhinovirus
	Respiratory syncytial virus
	Influenza virus
	Parainfluenza virus
	Human metapneuvirus
	Coronavirus
	Adenovirus
Atypical microorganisms	
	Mycoplasma pneumoniae
	Chlamydophila pneumoniae
	Legionella pneumophila
	Coxiella burnetii
Other	
	Sulphur dioxide (SO_2)
	Ozone (O_3)
	Nitrogen dioxide (NO_2)
	Particulate matter ($PM_{2,5}$, PM_{10})

Table 1. Most common causes of exacerbations of COPD.

4.3. Bacterial causes

Bacteria as cause of AECOPD are reported from 30% [48] up to 55% [27, 49]. The most common bacterial pathogens are *Streptococcus pneumoniae, Haemophilus influenzae, Moraxella catarrhalis* and in patients with more severe COPD also *Pseudomonas aeruginosa* [42, 48]. It is difficult to determine the role of bacteria in AECOPD, as 34-48% of patients with COPD are reported to be colonized with bacteria [26, 27, 50, 51]. Molecular typing of bacteria during exacerbations showed that the acquisition of new strains may cause exacerbations [52], but not every acquisition of a new strain is linked to an exacerbation.

4.4. Non-microbial causes

One tenth of AECOPD are due to environmental pollution, of which ozone, sulphur dioxide and nitrogen dioxide known and researched causes [53, 54]. Particulate matter (PM) is also related to increased admissions for COPD and other respiratory diseases [53, 55]. Particulate matter consists of a mixture of solid particles and liquid aerosols suspended in the air from natural sources, industrial activities and can also be traffic related [56]. Other possible, non-infectious causes may be left sided heart failure, change in environmental temperature, but about 30% of exacerbations are of unknown origin [6].

5. Clinical Presentation and Diagnosis

5.1. History

Patients with an AECOPD usually present with dyspnea, which may be acute but can also be a history of slowly progressive dyspnea. Coughing or sputum production may or may not be present. When expectorating sputum, it is important to assess whether sputum volume has increased and whether it is purulent (e.g. green). Purulent sputum is usually a sign of infection [57]. Fever or other signs of infection should be looked for. Hemoptysis may be present in case of a severe infection. Risk factors for atypical infections should be thought of.

5.2. Laboratory tests

Laboratory test can be performed if necessary. C-reactive protein as marker for inflammation can be performed. Additional laboratory tests can be performed depending on the differential diagnosis. If available, an arterial blood gas can be performed. Hypoxemia may be present and in more severe cases a patient can also retain CO_2. Hypercapnia is defined as arterial blood gas CO_2 (P_aCO_2) level above 45 mmHg (6,00 kPa) and hypercapnic respiratory failure as P_aCO_2 of >50 mmHg (6,67 kPa). When present it is important to assess if the hypercapnia is longer existing and to assess if the patient is being able to metabolically compensate the hypercapnia.

5.3. Radiology

A chest X-ray is mainly useful for excluding other pathology like pneumothorax, pleural fluid, congestive heart failure or otherwise. It may reveal consolidations or other pathology. In the acute phase a chest CT-scan has no additive value in the tract of diagnosing an exacerbation of COPD. It can be performed if doubts exist about the presence of pulmonary embolisms as an explanation for dyspnea and/or desaturation. In a patient with recurrent airways infections a CT-thorax can be performed to investigate whether bronchiectasis is present.

5.4. Biomarkers

Biomarkers can be used as indicators of a physiological state in which a patient is or may become, it can help in diagnosis, aetiology and prognosis. In theory, biomarkers could be used to predict exacerbations, to determine if a patient has increased inflammation, to distinguish type of inflammation (bacterial or viral infection or otherwise) or to predict clinical outcome after an AECOPD.

Many biomarkers have been researched of which many of them are of little clinical use. At this moment the most important biomarkers in AECOPD are CRP, serum IL-6, 8-isoprostane, H_2O_2 and procalcitonin (ProCT). These biomarkers are closely related to oxidative stress and inflammation. C-reactive protein is momentarily the most widely used marker of inflammation in clinical practice.

In patients with frequent exacerbations, both CRP and serum IL-6 levels are increased during a stable phase but also during the recovery period of an AECOPD [58, 59] compared to patients with infrequent exacerbations. Interleukin-6 is a cytokine which is widely expressed and produced in the body, and is not specific to the lung. Serum IL-6 has no additional value above CRP in clinical decision making. Interleukin-6 levels in sputum may be of use to predict therapy response [58], although more research is needed before clinical decisions can be made based on this biomarker. Similarly, there is a lack of studies which investigate the use of exhaled biomarkers 8-isoporstane and H_2O_2 for clinical purposes. Procalcitonin may be a biomarker which can discriminate in aetiology of an exacerbation but may also be used as therapeutic response parameter. Procalcitonin is the precursor of calcitonin and is released in response to a bacterial infection by many tissues under stimulation of several cytokines. Procalcitonin levels are minimally raised in viral infections [60], making it a relative specific diagnostic tool for bacterial infections. Most research has been performed in patients with community acquired pneumonia (CAP) [61]. It is suggested that ProCT could become a useful tool in clinical decision making regarding antibiotic therapy. There have been several trials to assess the utility of ProCT in AECOPD. In general ProCT-guided antibiotic therapy compared to standard management in AECOPD showed no differences in death from any cause, rates of intensive care unit (ICU) admission for any reason, duration of ICU stay, improvement of symptoms, difference in the quality-of-life score, re-exacerbation and readmission [62]. Procalcitonin-guided antibiotic therapy showed reduction in antibiotic prescription [62] and in one study [63] also reduction in antibiotic therapy duration, which in turn decreases the patient's exposure to antibiotics and related side effects, lowers the burden of antibiotic use and the risk of antimicrobial resistance. Procalcitonin is not yet being implemented in standard

http://dx.doi.org/10.5772/54867

care though, as it is relatively expensive and there has been little to no research performed outside Europe.

6. Management

The treatment of an AECOPD consists of supportive therapy, maximal bronchodilation, steroids to reduce the inflammation and treatment of the cause.

6.1. Supportive therapy

Oxygen delivery is one of the first supportive therapies which can be provided for a patient. Oxygen saturation should be at least 90% though in some cases lower saturations may also be accepted. Too much oxygen may cause hypercapnia as the drive to breathe in some COPD patients may rely on arterial O_2 pressure. Symptoms of acute hypercapnia are somnolence, headache, drowsiness, confusion, flushed skin or agitation. Physiotherapy during an admission for an AECOPD can prevent deterioration in skeletal muscle function and improve exercise capacity [64, 65]. Because an AECOPD is accompanied by an impaired energy balance due to a decreased dietary intake and an increased resting energy expenditure, nutritional support may also benefit the patient in terms of general well-being and prevention of muscle wasting [66-68].

6.2. Pharmacotherapy

An exacerbation is the result of increased inflammation causing increased flow limitation. Treatment should be directed towards controlling this exacerbated inflammation and maximizing bronchodilation. Short acting agents like salbutamol and ipratropium are mostly used for maximal bronchodilation, usually delivered by nebulizer. Many patients may not be able to generate the flows required to use other devices during an exacerbation. Corticosteroids have been proven to reduce time to recovery and treatment failure, increase FEV_1 and arterial hypoxemia [8]. Treatment schemes have been reported varying from 30 mg prednisolone orally to 60 mg intravenous, ranging from 5 days to two weeks. Studies showed that there is no difference in clinical outcome if a patient is treated with oral steroids compared to parenteral steroids [69]. Antibiotic treatment can be initiated when a bacterial infection is suspected. With the Anthonisen criteria [70] one can decide whether antibiotic treatment is necessary or not. These criteria are derived from a randomized placebo-controlled crossover trial which has been performed in the '80s where patients with COPD exacerbations were treated with antibiotics or placebo. The cardinal symptoms of infection in this study were increased sputum volume and purulence in combination with increased dyspnea. An exacerbation with all the previous 3 symptoms is called a type 1 exacerbation; two out of three symptoms have to be present for a type 2 exacerbation; one out of three and at least one other "minor symptom" (see table 2) have to be present for it to be a type 3 exacerbation. Patients with type 1 and type 2 exacerbations are most likely to benefit from antibiotic therapy. In Spain a pilot study was performed with hospitalized patients with AECOPD, where antibiotic therapy was given to patients with self-reported purulent sputum and withheld in patients with non-purulent sputum [71]. There was no difference between the two groups in treatment failure on day 3, suggesting patient reported non-purulent sputum may be a valid criterion to withhold antibiotics [71]. A Dutch study showed that addition of doxycycline to the treatment regimen with glucocorticoids of a patient with an exacerbation was superior on day 10 but equivalent on day 30 in terms of clinical success and clinical cure compared to glucocorticoids alone, even in patients not showing signs of infection [72]. Most recently Spanish investigators performed a multicenter trial where they suggested that treatment of a mild to moderate exacerbation with amoxicillin/clavulanate, independent of glucocorticoids treatment, might give better clinical cure after 10 days compared to placebo [73]. In this study the median time to next exacerbation was also increased in patients receiving antibiotics compared to placebo. Unfortunately, because of recruitment problems this study did not reach the calculated amount of patients needed, so that definite conclusions cannot be made from the results of this study.

Classification of AECOPD according to Anthonisen criteria	**Presence of symptoms and findings**
Type 1	Increased dyspnea Increased sputum volume Increased sputum purulence
Type 2	Two symptoms of type 1
Type 3	1 of three symptoms of type 1, plus at least one of the following findings: - Upper respiratory infection (sore throat, nasal discharge) within the past 5 days - Fever without other cause - Increased wheezing - Increased cough - Increase in respiratory rate or heart rate by 20% as compared with baseline

Table 2. Classification of acute exacerbations of COPD according to Anthonisen criteria [70]

7. Prevention

Preventing exacerbations is an important treatment goal in COPD. There is a wide range of preventive measures which have proven to reduce exacerbation frequency or hospitalization in patients with AECOPD.

7.1. Supportive measures

Influenza vaccination and pneumococcal vaccination have both been researched as preventive measures for infection associated exacerbations. Current GOLD guidelines [8] advise influenza vaccination for patients with COPD. Pneumococcal vaccination is mainly advised for elderly patients with COPD. Investigation on this subject is ongoing. Of the non-pharmacologic interventions, pulmonary rehabilitation is the most effective in reducing hospital admissions and mortality and improving health-related quality of life in COPD patients who have recently suffered an exacerbation of COPD [74].

7.2. Long-acting bronchodilators

Long-acting bronchodilators can be divided in two groups: long acting muscarinic receptor antagonists (LAMAs) and long acting β-agonists (LABAs). Both have proven to show a positive effect on exacerbation reduction and improvement in quality of life [75-79]. An overview of the long-acting bronchodilators is given in table 3.

LABA	LAMA
Formoterol	Tiotropium
Arfomoterol	Glycopyrronium
Salmeterol	
Indacaterol	

Table 3. An overview of available long-acting bronchodilators.

Of the long-acting bronchodilators, indacaterol and glycopyrronium are the most recent additions for the treatment of COPD. Indacaterol is proven to be superior to formoterol, salmeterol and tiotropium in terms of use of rescue medication, dyspnoea score and health related quality of life. Compared to salmeterol and formoterol it is also superior in improving spirometry values. Indacaterol is non-inferior to tiotropium but when added to tiotropium therapy it is superior compared to tiotropium alone [80]. Indacaterol also lowers the risk of AECOPD compared to placebo [78, 81, 82]. Glycopyrronium has been approved in 2012 as therapy for COPD. It provides significant improvements in lung function, dyspnoea, health status, exacerbation frequency and rescue medication use versus placebo, and is comparable to tiotropium [83, 84]. The combination of glycopyrronium and indacaterol has shown superiority in bronchodilation compared to indacaterol alone [85]. Glycopyrronium has not been compared to other LABAs yet.

7.3. Inhalation corticosteroids

Inhalation corticosteroids (ICS) can be given to patients with high risk of exacerbations. In several studies ICS provided a reduction of symptoms (dyspnea, cough) and reduced the frequency of exacerbations [86-88]. The GOLD guidelines advise treatment for high exacerbation risk patients with few symptoms (group C) with a combination of ICS/LABA or a LAMA alone, or a combination of LABA and LAMA [8]. For high exacerbation risk patients who have many symptoms (group D) the same treatment is advised as for group C, also a combination of all three classes of inhalation drugs is possible [8].

7.4. Phosphodiesterase inhibitors

Currently, two phosphodiesterase inhibitors are available for the treatment of COPD: theophylline and roflumilast. Theophylline is a xanthine derivative which acts as a non-selective phosphodiesterase inhibitor. It has bronchodilator effects, improves symptoms and there is evidence that it can reduce exacerbations [89-91]. It is a drug which needs therapeutic window monitoring. It can interact with many drugs and can have toxic side effects which may be potentially dangerous, like cardiac arrhythmia. Therapy with theophyllines is not recommended if LABAs are available but can be used as add-on therapy [8]. Roflumilast is a selective phosphodiesterase-4 inhibitor. It increases prebronchodilator FEV1 and can reduce exacerbations in a selected group of patients with COPD [92, 93]. In all trials patients in the roflumilast group experienced more side effects in comparison to patients in the placebo groups. The side effects were mostly gastro-intestinal related (nausea, diarrhoea, weight loss) and headache. These adverse events were associated with increased patient withdrawal in the roflumilast groups. The design of the trials limits the generalizability of these results. The included COPD patients were required to have symptoms of chronic bronchitis and AECOPD in the past. More investigation is needed to determine the exact place of this medication in the treatment of AECOPD.

7.5. Macrolide antibiotics

Antibiotic prevention of exacerbations is a highly researched topic in COPD. The most promising class of antibiotics appear to be macrolides. In various chronic lung diseases they seem to have an immune modulatory function.

7.5.1. Proposed working mechanism

Much *in vivo* and *in vitro* research has been performed with macrolide antibiotics. The effects of macrolides can be divided in antimicrobial effects and immune modulatory effects. Macrolides bind to the 50S subunit of the bacterial ribosome and inhibit bacterial protein synthesis [94]. Most macrolides have a uniform degree of activity; their antimicrobial spectrum extends from Gram-positive bacteria to a limited activity against Gram-negative bacteria [95]. Of the macrolides, azithromycin displays superior activity against Gram-negative organisms, such as *H. influenzae* [94]. Compared to other macrolides as erythromycin and clarithromycin, azithromycin also has better uptake in peripheral blood polymorphonuclear neutrophils (PMN) with slower release [96, 97], better tissue uptake and tissue concentrations are higher long after the last administered dose [98, 99]. *Pseudomonas aeruginosa* is a Gram-negative rod which has intrinsic resistance for macrolides but has nonetheless been extensively studied in combination with macrolides. Studies have shown that macrolides influence the virulence of not only *P. aeruginosa* [100-102] but also other microorganisms, like *Proteus mirabilis* [103], *Salmonella enterica* [104], *Staphylococcus epidermidis* [105] and *H. influenzae* [106]. Macrolides alter the biofilm around bacteria [105-107], in *P. aeruginosa* this may facilitate phagocytosis by PMN [101]. It is also suggested that macrolides block quorum sensing [108, 109] in *P. aeruginosa,* reduce flagellin synthesis and expression [103, 104] and reduce production of bacterial exoenzymes [100]. In murine models and in in vitro studies macrolides have shown to influence respiratory viral infections. In one study therapy with erythromycin increased survival rates in mice infected with lethal doses of influenza virus [110]. This effect might be exerted through the inhibitory action of erythromycin against virus-induced inflammatory responses in the lung. The production of interferon-gamma (IFN-γ) in the lungs was significantly decreased by the administration of erythromycin to the infected mice. Two in vitro studies researching the effect of erythromycin and clarithromycin in human tracheal cells infected with rhinovirus and influenza A virus, also showed that macrolides decrease the production of pro-inflammatory cytokines and inhibited activation of nuclear factor-κB (a regulating factor in transcription of DNA in response to cellular stress) [111, 112]. These antiviral effects of macrolides have not yet been proven in patients, although there is evidence that macrolides may prevent common colds which are mostly of viral aetiology [113]. Macrolides support the airway innate immune system by maintaining airway epithelial integrity [114, 115]. In vitro [116] and in vivo [117] studies show that macrolides improve alveolar macrophage phagocytosis function. Macrolide therapy stimulates the prolonged degranulation of neutrophils (suggesting anti-inflammatory activity in non-infective inflammation), decreases long term oxidative burst and can decrease the release of pro-inflammatory cytokines (such as IL-6 and IL-8) in healthy individuals [118]. In vitro it is observed that macrolides decrease the release of IL-1β, IL-6 and tumor necrosis factor-alpha (TNF-α) in sputum cells of patients with COPD [119]. Azithromycin exerts direct inhibitory effects on mucus secretion from airway epithelial cells in vitro and in vivo [120].

7.5.2. Success of macrolides in chronic lung diseases

Diffuse panbronchiolitis is a progressive inflammatory disorder of the airways found almost exclusively in Japan. Clinically it is characterized by chronic cough, excessive sputum production, exertional breathlessness, chronic sinusitis and Pseudomonas colonization [121]. Untreated, the prognosis of diffuse panbronchiolitis is poor, with progressive deterioration of lung function, the development of diffuse bronchiectasis and death caused by respiratory failure. The introduction of long-term macrolide therapy has resulted in dramatic improvements in survival, with 5-year survival rates increasing from 63 to 92% [121, 122]. Significant symptom reduction and improved pulmonary function have also been achieved [123-126]. Also in patients with cystic fibrosis (CF) who are colonized with *P. aeruginosa,* macrolide therapy had led to improvement in FEV_1 and forced vital capacity (FVC), a reduction in exacerbation rate, a reduction in hospital days and days of intravenous antibiotic use, delaying time until the first exacerbation and reducing number of additional courses of antibiotics [127-132]. A Cochrane review of macrolide therapy concluded that treatment with azithromycin had a small but significant effect on pulmonary function in patients with cystic fibrosis [133]. In a in New Zealand performed randomized controlled trial in non-CF bronchiectasis, maintenance treatment with 3 times a week 500 mg azithromycin showed a reduction in exacerbations [134] though no effects were seen in quality of life and lung function. In a Dutch study where a treatment scheme was given with daily 250 mg azithromycin, the reduction in exacerbations was accompanied by an improved quality of life assessed by St George's Respiratory Questionnaire (SGRQ) and an increase in lung function [135]. As for COPD there have been few researches concerning macrolides in preventing AECOPD. One published study has examined the effect of clarithromycin treatment in COPD [136]. This was a prospective double-blind randomized controlled trial of 67 patients with moderately severe COPD. The effects of 3 months' clarithromycin therapy on health status, exacerbation rate and sputum bacterial numbers were measured. Overall, no significant benefit was seen in any measure. However, significant improvements in both the SGRQ symptom score and 36-item short-form health survey (SF-36) physical function score were seen. A Japanese study performed in 1997 investigated the effect of long-term erythromycin therapy on common colds in patients with COPD [113]. It was a prospective, randomized, controlled but not blinded study. Patients who received erythromycin therapy had less common colds and less subsequent AECOPD compared to patients in the control group. In 2006, another study had been performed in the UK to investigate the influence of erythromycin on exacerbation of COPD [137]. Unfortunately, the total number of patients needed for inclusion was not reached. Although the study showed a significant reduction in number of exacerbations in COPD patients who received 1 year daily erythromycin, the reached conclusions should be carefully interpreted. The most recent study published concerning long term macrolide therapy in COPD was performed in the USA with over 1,000 patients. It showed a reduction in time to first exacerbation and a reduced risk for exacerbations in patients receiving daily azithromycin during 1 year [138]. The study participants were patients who had at least 1 treated exacerbation in the previous year or who were on continuous supplemental oxygen or had an emergency department (ED) visit or hospital admission for an exacerbation COPD. The applicability of these results is somewhat difficult. The results of the study could suggest that long term azithromycin can be given to many COPD patients, even to those who are not actually frequent exacerbators. The place of azithromycin in the prevention of COPD exacerbations is a topic which needs further research.

7.5.3. Antimicrobial resistance

Giving long term antibiotic treatment to a patient may have consequences; the development of antimicrobial resistance is by far the most important one. Several researches have shown that the erm(B) and mef genes are mostly responsible for macrolide resistance in streptococci bacteria [139-142]. This resistance can develop even when short term therapy with macrolides is given [141]. The participants receiving azithromycin in the USA study, where a 1-year therapy was administered, were less likely to be colonized with respiratory pathogens but more likely to become colonized with macrolide resistant pathogens [138]. In the UK study in patients with COPD the researchers found there were no significant changes in resistance of sputum pathogens (*H. influenzae, S. pneumoniae, M. catarrhalis*) after 1 year of daily erythromycin [137]. In a Dutch study investigating antibiotic treatment before cardiovascular surgery 300 patients were treated with 2 weeks of clarithromycin. A significant rise in macrolide resistance in oropharyngeal flora was observed and this resistance continued to exist for at least 8 weeks [140]. Since macrolide resistance in pneumococci is already a known problem [141, 143, 144] it is of great importance to prevent the development of resistance in other microorganisms.

Author details

S. Uzun[1], R.S. Djamin[1], H.C. Hoogsteden[2], J.G.J.V. Aerts[1,2] and M.M. van der Eerden[2]

1 Department of Respiratory Medicine, Amphia Ziekenhuis, Breda, The Netherlands

2 Department of Respiratory Medicine, Erasmus Medical Centre, Rotterdam, The Netherlands

References

[1] Pauwels, R, et al. COPD exacerbations: the importance of a standard definition. Respir Med, (2004)., 99-107.

[2] Rabe, K. F, et al. Global strategy for the diagnosis, management, and prevention of chronic obstructive pulmonary disease: GOLD executive summary. Am J Respir Crit Care Med, (2007)., 532-555.

[3] Seemungal, T. A, et al. Effect of exacerbation on quality of life in patients with chronic obstructive pulmonary disease. Am J Respir Crit Care Med, (1998). Pt 1): , 1418-1422.

[4] Donaldson, G. C, et al. Relationship between exacerbation frequency and lung function decline in chronic obstructive pulmonary disease. Thorax, (2002)., 847-852.

[5] Terzano, C, et al. Comorbidity, hospitalization, and mortality in COPD: results from a longitudinal study. Lung, (2010)., 321-329.

[6] Connors, A. F, et al. Outcomes following acute exacerbation of severe chronic obstructive lung disease. The SUPPORT investigators (Study to Understand Prognoses and Preferences for Outcomes and Risks of Treatments). Am J Respir Crit Care Med, (1996). Pt 1): , 959-967.

[7] Mathers, C, & Ma, B. T. Fat D, Global Burden of Disease: 2004 update, (2008). World Health Organization. , 146.

[8] Vestbo, J. Global strategy for the diagnosis, management, and prevention of chronic obstructive pulmonary disease (revised 2011), (2011). Global Initiative for Chronic Obstructive Lung Disease. , 78.

[9] Buist, A. S, Vollmer, W. M, & Mcburnie, M. A. Worldwide burden of COPD in high- and low-income countries. Part I. The burden of obstructive lung disease (BOLD) initiative. Int J Tuberc Lung Dis, (2008)., 703-708.

[10] Salvi, S. S, & Barnes, P. J. Chronic obstructive pulmonary disease in non-smokers. Lancet, (2009)., 733-743.

[11] Atsou, K, Chouaid, C, & Hejblum, G. Variability of the chronic obstructive pulmonary disease key epidemiological data in Europe: systematic review. BMC Med, (2011). , 7.

[12] Rycroft, C. E, et al. Epidemiology of chronic obstructive pulmonary disease: a literature review. Int J Chron Obstruct Pulmon Dis, (2012). , 457-494.

[13] Langsetmo, L, et al. Underreporting exacerbation of chronic obstructive pulmonary disease in a longitudinal cohort. Am J Respir Crit Care Med, (2008). , 396-401.

[14] Seemungal, T. A, et al. Time course and recovery of exacerbations in patients with chronic obstructive pulmonary disease. Am J Respir Crit Care Med, (2000). , 1608-1613.

[15] Jenkins, C. R, et al. Seasonality and determinants of moderate and severe COPD exacerbations in the TORCH study. Eur Respir J, (2012). , 38-45.

[16] Hurst, J. R, et al. Temporal clustering of exacerbations in chronic obstructive pulmonary disease. Am J Respir Crit Care Med, (2009). , 369-374.

[17] Hurst, J. R, et al. Susceptibility to exacerbation in chronic obstructive pulmonary disease. N Engl J Med, (2010). , 1128-1138.

[18] Ito, K, et al. Depression, but not sleep disorder, is an independent factor affecting exacerbations and hospitalization in patients with chronic obstructive pulmonary disease. Respirology, (2012). , 940-949.

[19] Papaioannou, A. I, et al. The impact of depressive symptoms on recovery and outcome of hospitalised COPD exacerbations. Eur Respir J, (2012).

[20] Cosio, M. G, Saetta, M, & Agusti, A. Immunologic aspects of chronic obstructive pulmonary disease. N Engl J Med, (2009). , 2445-2454.

[21] Baines, K. J, Simpson, J. L, & Gibson, P. G. Innate immune responses are increased in chronic obstructive pulmonary disease. PLoS One, (2011). , e18426.

[22] Hogg, J. C, et al. The nature of small-airway obstruction in chronic obstructive pulmonary disease. N Engl J Med, (2004). , 2645-2653.

[23] Keatings, V. M, et al. Differences in interleukin-8 and tumor necrosis factor-alpha in induced sputum from patients with chronic obstructive pulmonary disease or asthma. Am J Respir Crit Care Med, (1996). , 530-534.

[24] Sethi, S, & Murphy, T. F. Infection in the pathogenesis and course of chronic obstructive pulmonary disease. N Engl J Med, (2008). , 2355-2365.

[25] Marin, A, et al. Effect of Bronchial Colonisation on Airway and Systemic Inflammation in Stable COPD. COPD, (2012).

[26] Wilkinson, T. M, et al. Effect of interactions between lower airway bacterial and rhinoviral infection in exacerbations of COPD. Chest, (2006). , 317-324.

[27] Papi, A, et al. Infections and airway inflammation in chronic obstructive pulmonary disease severe exacerbations. Am J Respir Crit Care Med, (2006). , 1114-1121.

[28] Bhowmik, A, et al. Relation of sputum inflammatory markers to symptoms and lung function changes in COPD exacerbations. Thorax, (2000). , 114-120.

[29] Tsoumakidou, M, et al. Nitrosative stress, heme oxygenase-1 expression and airway inflammation during severe exacerbations of COPD. Chest, (2005). , 1911-1918.

[30] Hurst, J. R, et al. Systemic and upper and lower airway inflammation at exacerbation of chronic obstructive pulmonary disease. Am J Respir Crit Care Med, (2006). , 71-78.

[31] Gerritsen, W. B, et al. Markers of inflammation and oxidative stress in exacerbated chronic obstructive pulmonary disease patients. Respir Med, (2005). , 84-90.

[32] Yamamoto, K, & Rose-john, S. Therapeutic blockade of interleukin-6 in chronic inflammatory disease. Clin Pharmacol Ther, (2012). , 574-576.

[33] Chung, K. F. Cytokines in chronic obstructive pulmonary disease. Eur Respir J Suppl, (2001). , 50s-59s.

[34] Smith, W. B, et al. Interleukin-8 induces neutrophil transendothelial migration. Immunology, (1991). , 65-72.

[35] Sinden, N. J, & Stockley, R. A. Systemic inflammation and comorbidity in COPD: a result of'overspill' of inflammatory mediators from the lungs? Review of the evidence. Thorax, (2010). , 930-936.

[36] Dekhuijzen, P. N, et al. Increased exhalation of hydrogen peroxide in patients with stable and unstable chronic obstructive pulmonary disease. Am J Respir Crit Care Med, (1996). Pt 1): , 813-816.

[37] Antczak, A, et al. Exhaled eicosanoids and biomarkers of oxidative stress in exacerbation of chronic obstructive pulmonary disease. Arch Med Sci, (2012). , 277-285.

[38] Biernacki, W. A, Kharitonov, S. A, & Barnes, P. J. Increased leukotriene B4 and 8-isoprostane in exhaled breath condensate of patients with exacerbations of COPD. Thorax, (2003). , 294-298.

[39] Maestrelli, P, et al. Decreased haem oxygenase-1 and increased inducible nitric oxide synthase in the lung of severe COPD patients. Eur Respir J, (2003). , 971-976.

[40] Maestrelli, P, et al. Increased expression of heme oxygenase (HO)-1 in alveolar spaces and HO-2 in alveolar walls of smokers. Am J Respir Crit Care Med, (2001). Pt 1): , 1508-1513.

[41] Sapey, E, & Stockley, R. A. COPD exacerbations. 2: aetiology. Thorax, (2006). , 250-258.

[42] Wedzicha, J. A, & Seemungal, T. A. COPD exacerbations: defining their cause and prevention. Lancet, (2007). , 786-796.

[43] Fisman, D. Seasonality of viral infections: mechanisms and unknowns. Clin Microbiol Infect, (2012). , 946-954.

[44] Mallia, P, et al. Experimental rhinovirus infection as a human model of chronic obstructive pulmonary disease exacerbation. Am J Respir Crit Care Med, (2011). , 734-742.

[45] Seemungal, T, et al. Respiratory viruses, symptoms, and inflammatory markers in acute exacerbations and stable chronic obstructive pulmonary disease. Am J Respir Crit Care Med, (2001). , 1618-1623.

[46] Rohde, G, et al. Respiratory viruses in exacerbations of chronic obstructive pulmonary disease requiring hospitalisation: a case-control study. Thorax, (2003). , 37-42.

[47] Ko, F. W, et al. Viral etiology of acute exacerbations of COPD in Hong Kong. Chest, (2007). , 900-908.

[48] Ko, F. W, et al. A 1-year prospective study of the infectious etiology in patients hospitalized with acute exacerbations of COPD. Chest, (2007). , 44-52.

[49] Bafadhel, M, et al. Acute exacerbations of chronic obstructive pulmonary disease: identification of biologic clusters and their biomarkers. Am J Respir Crit Care Med, (2011). , 662-671.

[50] Sethi, S, et al. Airway inflammation and bronchial bacterial colonization in chronic obstructive pulmonary disease. Am J Respir Crit Care Med, (2006). , 991-998.

[51] Zhang, M, et al. Relevance of lower airway bacterial colonization, airway inflammation, and pulmonary function in the stable stage of chronic obstructive pulmonary disease. Eur J Clin Microbiol Infect Dis, (2010). , 1487-1493.

[52] Sethi, S, et al. New strains of bacteria and exacerbations of chronic obstructive pulmonary disease. N Engl J Med, (2002). , 465-471.

[53] Ko, F. W, et al. Temporal relationship between air pollutants and hospital admissions for chronic obstructive pulmonary disease in Hong Kong. Thorax, (2007). , 780-705.

[54] Sint, T, Donohue, J. F, & Ghio, A. J. Ambient air pollution particles and the acute exacerbation of chronic obstructive pulmonary disease. Inhal Toxicol, (2008). , 25-29.

[55] Qiu, H, et al. Effects of coarse particulate matter on emergency hospital admissions for respiratory diseases: a time-series analysis in Hong Kong. Environ Health Perspect, (2012). , 572-576.

[56] Valavanidis, A, Fiotakis, K, & Vlachogianni, T. Airborne particulate matter and human health: toxicological assessment and importance of size and composition of particles for oxidative damage and carcinogenic mechanisms. J Environ Sci Health C Environ Carcinog Ecotoxicol Rev, (2008). , 339-362.

[57] Stockley, R. A, et al. Relationship of sputum color to nature and outpatient management of acute exacerbations of COPD. Chest, (2000). , 1638-1645.

[58] Perera, W. R, et al. Inflammatory changes, recovery and recurrence at COPD exacerbation. Eur Respir J, (2007). , 527-534.

[59] Agusti, A, et al. Persistent systemic inflammation is associated with poor clinical outcomes in COPD: a novel phenotype. PLoS One, (2012). , e37483.

[60] Linscheid, P, et al. In vitro and in vivo calcitonin I gene expression in parenchymal cells: a novel product of human adipose tissue. Endocrinology, (2003). , 5578-5584.

[61] Schuetz, P, Amin, D. N, & Greenwald, J. L. Role of procalcitonin in managing adult patients with respiratory tract infections. Chest, (2012). , 1063-1073.

[62] Tokman, S, Schuetz, P, & Bent, S. Procalcitonin-guided antibiotic therapy for chronic obstructive pulmonary disease exacerbations. Expert Rev Anti Infect Ther, (2011). , 727-735.

[63] Schuetz, P, et al. Effect of procalcitonin-based guidelines vs standard guidelines on antibiotic use in lower respiratory tract infections: the ProHOSP randomized controlled trial. JAMA, (2009). , 1059-1066.

[64] Troosters, T, et al. Resistance training prevents deterioration in quadriceps muscle function during acute exacerbations of chronic obstructive pulmonary disease. Am J Respir Crit Care Med, (2010). , 1072-1077.

[65] Kirsten, D. K, et al. Exercise training improves recovery in patients with COPD after an acute exacerbation. Respir Med, (1998). , 1191-1118.

[66] Vermeeren, M. A, Schols, A. M, & Wouters, E. F. Effects of an acute exacerbation on nutritional and metabolic profile of patients with COPD. Eur Respir J, (1997). , 2264-2269.

[67] Vermeeren, M. A, et al. Nutritional support in patients with chronic obstructive pulmonary disease during hospitalization for an acute exacerbation; a randomized controlled feasibility trial. Clin Nutr, (2004). , 1184-1192.

[68] Saudny-unterberger, H, Martin, J. G, & Gray-donald, K. Impact of nutritional support on functional status during an acute exacerbation of chronic obstructive pulmonary disease. Am J Respir Crit Care Med, (1997). Pt 1): , 794-799.

[69] De Jong, Y. P, et al. Oral or IV prednisolone in the treatment of COPD exacerbations: a randomized, controlled, double-blind study. Chest, (2007). , 1741-1747.

[70] Anthonisen, N. R, et al. Antibiotic therapy in exacerbations of chronic obstructive pulmonary disease. Ann Intern Med, (1987). , 196-204.

[71] Soler, N, et al. Sputum purulence-guided antibiotic use in hospitalised patients with exacerbations of COPD. Eur Respir J, (2012).

[72] Daniels, J. M, et al. Antibiotics in addition to systemic corticosteroids for acute exacerbations of chronic obstructive pulmonary disease. Am J Respir Crit Care Med, (2010). , 150-157.

[73] Llor, C, et al. Efficacy of Antibiotic Therapy for Acute Exacerbations of Mild to Moderate COPD. Am J Respir Crit Care Med, (2012).

[74] Puhan, M. A, et al. Pulmonary rehabilitation following exacerbations of chronic obstructive pulmonary disease. Cochrane Database Syst Rev, (2011). , CD005305.

[75] Donohue, J. F, et al. A 6-month, placebo-controlled study comparing lung function and health status changes in COPD patients treated with tiotropium or salmeterol. Chest, (2002). , 47-55.

[76] Casaburi, R, et al. A long-term evaluation of once-daily inhaled tiotropium in chronic obstructive pulmonary disease. Eur Respir J, (2002). , 217-224.

[77] Tashkin, D. P, et al. A 4-year trial of tiotropium in chronic obstructive pulmonary disease. N Engl J Med, (2008). , 1543-1554.

[78] Chapman, K. R, et al. Long-term safety and efficacy of indacaterol, a long-acting beta(2)-agonist, in subjects with COPD: a randomized, placebo-controlled study. Chest, (2011). , 68-75.

[79] Stockley, R. A, Chopra, N, & Rice, L. Addition of salmeterol to existing treatment in patients with COPD: a 12 month study. Thorax, (2006). , 122-128.

[80] Mckeage, K. Indacaterol: a review of its use as maintenance therapy in patients with chronic obstructive pulmonary disease. Drugs, (2012). , 543-563.

[81] Donohue, J. F, et al. Once-daily bronchodilators for chronic obstructive pulmonary disease: indacaterol versus tiotropium. Am J Respir Crit Care Med, (2010). , 155-162.

[82] Dahl, R, et al. Efficacy of a new once-daily long-acting inhaled beta2-agonist indacaterol versus twice-daily formoterol in COPD. Thorax, (2010). , 473-479.

[83] Urzo, D, et al. Efficacy and safety of once-daily NVA237 in patients with moderate-to-severe COPD: the GLOW1 trial. Respir Res, (2011). , 156.

[84] Kerwin, E, et al. Efficacy and safety of NVA237 versus placebo and tiotropium in patients with COPD: the GLOW2 study. Eur Respir J, (2012). , 1106-1114.

[85] Van Noord, J. A, et al. QVA149 demonstrates superior bronchodilation compared with indacaterol or placebo in patients with chronic obstructive pulmonary disease. Thorax, (2010). , 1086-1091.

[86] Calverley, P. M, et al. Salmeterol and fluticasone propionate and survival in chronic obstructive pulmonary disease. N Engl J Med, (2007). , 775-789.

[87] Wedzicha, J. A, et al. The prevention of chronic obstructive pulmonary disease exacerbations by salmeterol/fluticasone propionate or tiotropium bromide. Am J Respir Crit Care Med, (2008). , 19-26.

[88] Jones, P. W, et al. Disease severity and the effect of fluticasone propionate on chronic obstructive pulmonary disease exacerbations. Eur Respir J, (2003). , 68-73.

[89] Zhou, Y, et al. Positive benefits of theophylline in a randomized, double-blind, parallel-group, placebo-controlled study of low-dose, slow-release theophylline in the treatment of COPD for 1 year. Respirology, (2006). , 603-610.

[90] Rossi, A, et al. Comparison of the efficacy, tolerability, and safety of formoterol dry powder and oral, slow-release theophylline in the treatment of COPD. Chest, (2002). , 1058-1069.

[91] ZuWallackR.L., et al., Salmeterol plus theophylline combination therapy in the treatment of COPD. Chest, (2001). , 1661-1670.

[92] Calverley, P. M, et al. Roflumilast in symptomatic chronic obstructive pulmonary disease: two randomised clinical trials. Lancet, (2009). , 685-694.

[93] Fabbri, L. M, et al. Roflumilast in moderate-to-severe chronic obstructive pulmonary disease treated with longacting bronchodilators: two randomised clinical trials. Lancet, (2009). , 695-703.

[94] Retsema, J, et al. Spectrum and mode of action of azithromycin (CP-62,993), a new 15-membered-ring macrolide with improved potency against gram-negative organisms. Antimicrob Agents Chemother, (1987). , 1939-1947.

[95] Williams, J. D, & Sefton, A. M. Comparison of macrolide antibiotics. J Antimicrob Chemother, (1993). Suppl C: , 11-26.

[96] Bosnar, M, et al. Cellular uptake and efflux of azithromycin, erythromycin, clarithromycin, telithromycin, and cethromycin. Antimicrob Agents Chemother, (2005). , 2372-2377.

[97] Fietta, A, & Merlini, C. and G. Gialdroni Grassi, Requirements for intracellular accumulation and release of clarithromycin and azithromycin by human phagocytes. J Chemother, (1997). , 23-31.

[98] Foulds, G, Shepard, R. M, & Johnson, R. B. The pharmacokinetics of azithromycin in human serum and tissues. J Antimicrob Chemother, (1990). Suppl A: , 73-82.

[99] Girard, A. E, et al. Pharmacokinetic and in vivo studies with azithromycin (CP-62,993), a new macrolide with an extended half-life and excellent tissue distribution. Antimicrob Agents Chemother, (1987). , 1948-1954.

[100] Mizukane, R, et al. Comparative in vitro exoenzyme-suppressing activities of azithromycin and other macrolide antibiotics against Pseudomonas aeruginosa. Antimicrob Agents Chemother, (1994). , 528-533.

[101] Takeoka, K, et al. The in vitro effect of macrolides on the interaction of human polymorphonuclear leukocytes with Pseudomonas aeruginosa in biofilm. Chemotherapy, (1998). , 190-197.

[102] Tateda, K, et al. Potential of macrolide antibiotics to inhibit protein synthesis of Pseudomonas aeruginosa: suppression of virulence factors and stress response. J Infect Chemother, (2000). , 1-7.

[103] Kawamura-sato, K, et al. Postantibiotic suppression effect of macrolides on the expression of flagellin in Pseudomonas aeruginosa and Proteus mirabilis. J Infect Chemother, (2001). , 51-54.

[104] Matsui, H, et al. Azithromycin inhibits the formation of flagellar filaments without suppressing flagellin synthesis in Salmonella enterica serovar typhimurium. Antimicrob Agents Chemother, (2005). , 3396-3403.

[105] Yasuda, H, et al. Interaction between clarithromycin and biofilms formed by Staphylococcus epidermidis. Antimicrob Agents Chemother, (1994). , 138-141.

[106] Starner, T. D, et al. Subinhibitory concentrations of azithromycin decrease nontypeable Haemophilus influenzae biofilm formation and Diminish established biofilms. Antimicrob Agents Chemother, (2008). , 137-145.

[107] Ichimiya, T, et al. The influence of azithromycin on the biofilm formation of Pseudomonas aeruginosa in vitro. Chemotherapy, (1996). , 186-191.

[108] Skindersoe, M. E, et al. Effects of antibiotics on quorum sensing in Pseudomonas aeruginosa. Antimicrob Agents Chemother, (2008). , 3648-3663.

[109] Molinari, G, et al. Inhibition of Pseudomonas aeruginosa virulence factors by subinhibitory concentrations of azithromycin and other macrolide antibiotics. J Antimicrob Chemother, (1993). , 681-688.

[110] Sato, K, et al. Therapeutic effect of erythromycin on influenza virus-induced lung injury in mice. Am J Respir Crit Care Med, (1998). Pt 1): , 853-857.

[111] Suzuki, T, et al. Erythromycin inhibits rhinovirus infection in cultured human tracheal epithelial cells. Am J Respir Crit Care Med, (2002). , 1113-1118.

[112] Yamaya, M, et al. Clarithromycin inhibits type a seasonal influenza virus infection in human airway epithelial cells. J Pharmacol Exp Ther, (2010). , 81-90.

[113] Suzuki, T, et al. Erythromycin and common cold in COPD. Chest, (2001). , 730-733.

[114] Halldorsson, S, et al. Azithromycin maintains airway epithelial integrity during Pseudomonas aeruginosa infection. Am J Respir Cell Mol Biol, (2010). , 62-68.

[115] Asgrimsson, V, et al. Novel effects of azithromycin on tight junction proteins in human airway epithelia. Antimicrob Agents Chemother, (2006). , 1805-1812.

[116] Hodge, S, et al. Azithromycin improves macrophage phagocytic function and expression of mannose receptor in chronic obstructive pulmonary disease. Am J Respir Crit Care Med, (2008). , 139-148.

[117] Hodge, S, et al. Azithromycin increases phagocytosis of apoptotic bronchial epithelial cells by alveolar macrophages. Eur Respir J, (2006). , 486-495.

[118] Culic, O, et al. Azithromycin modulates neutrophil function and circulating inflammatory mediators in healthy human subjects. Eur J Pharmacol, (2002). , 277-289.

[119] Marjanovic, N, et al. Macrolide antibiotics broadly and distinctively inhibit cytokine and chemokine production by COPD sputum cells in vitro. Pharmacol Res, (2011). , 389-397.

[120] Shimizu, T, & Shimizu, S. Azithromycin inhibits mucus hypersecretion from airway epithelial cells. Mediators Inflamm, 2012. (2012). , 265714.

[121] Kudoh, S. Applying lessons learned in the treatment of diffuse panbronchiolitis to other chronic inflammatory diseases. Am J Med, (2004). Suppl 9A: , 12S-19S.

[122] Kudoh, S, et al. Improvement of survival in patients with diffuse panbronchiolitis treated with low-dose erythromycin. Am J Respir Crit Care Med, (1998). Pt 1): , 1829-1832.

[123] Fujii, T, et al. Long term effect of erythromycin therapy in patients with chronic Pseudomonas aeruginosa infection. Thorax, (1995). , 1246-1252.

[124] Ichikawa, Y, et al. Reversible airway lesions in diffuse panbronchiolitis. Detection by high-resolution computed tomography. Chest, (1995). , 120-125.

[125] Kadota, J, et al. Long-term efficacy and safety of clarithromycin treatment in patients with diffuse panbronchiolitis. Respir Med, (2003). , 844-850.

[126] Shirai, T, Sato, A, & Chida, K. Effect of 14-membered ring macrolide therapy on chronic respiratory tract infections and polymorphonuclear leukocyte activity. Intern Med, (1995). , 469-474.

[127] Clement, A, et al. Long term effects of azithromycin in patients with cystic fibrosis: A double blind, placebo controlled trial. Thorax, (2006). , 895-902.

[128] Hansen, C. R, et al. Long-term azitromycin treatment of cystic fibrosis patients with chronic Pseudomonas aeruginosa infection; an observational cohort study. J Cyst Fibros, (2005). , 35-40.

[129] Saiman, L, et al. Azithromycin in patients with cystic fibrosis chronically infected with Pseudomonas aeruginosa: a randomized controlled trial. JAMA, (2003). , 1749-1756.

[130] Pirzada, O. M, et al. Improved lung function and body mass index associated with long-term use of Macrolide antibiotics. J Cyst Fibros, (2003). , 69-71.

[131] Equi, A, et al. Long term azithromycin in children with cystic fibrosis: a randomised, placebo-controlled crossover trial. Lancet, (2002). , 978-984.

[132] Wolter, J, et al. Effect of long term treatment with azithromycin on disease parameters in cystic fibrosis: a randomised trial. Thorax, (2002). , 212-216.

[133] Southern, K. W, Barker, P. M, & Solis, A. Macrolide antibiotics for cystic fibrosis. Cochrane Database Syst Rev, (2004). , CD002203.

[134] Wong, C, et al. Azithromycin for prevention of exacerbations in non-cystic fibrosis bronchiectasis (EMBRACE): a randomised, double-blind, placebo-controlled trial. Lancet, (2012). , 660-667.

[135] Altenburg, J, De Graaff, C, Van Der Werf, T, & Boersma, W. Long term azithromycin treatment: A randomised placebo-controlled trial in non-CF bronchiectasis; results from the BAT trial in European Respiratory Society Congress (2011). Amsterdam.

[136] Banerjee, D, Khair, O. A, & Honeybourne, D. The effect of oral clarithromycin on health status and sputum bacteriology in stable COPD. Respir Med, (2005). , 208-215.

[137] Seemungal, T. A, et al. Long-term erythromycin therapy is associated with decreased chronic obstructive pulmonary disease exacerbations. Am J Respir Crit Care Med, (2008). , 1139-1147.

[138] Albert, R. K, et al. Azithromycin for Prevention of Exacerbations of COPD. N Engl J Med, (2011). , 689-698.

[139] Shortridge, V. D, et al. Prevalence of macrolide resistance mechanisms in Streptococcus pneumoniae isolates from a multicenter antibiotic resistance surveillance study conducted in the United States in 1994-1995. Clin Infect Dis, (1999). , 1186-1188.

[140] Berg, H. F, et al. Emergence and persistence of macrolide resistance in oropharyngeal flora and elimination of nasal carriage of Staphylococcus aureus after therapy with slow-release clarithromycin: a randomized, double-blind, placebo-controlled study. Antimicrob Agents Chemother, (2004). , 4183-4188.

[141] Malhotra-kumar, S, et al. Effect of azithromycin and clarithromycin therapy on pharyngeal carriage of macrolide-resistant streptococci in healthy volunteers: a randomised, double-blind, placebo-controlled study. Lancet, (2007). , 482-490.

[142] Leclercq, R, & Courvalin, P. Resistance to macrolides and related antibiotics in Streptococcus pneumoniae. Antimicrob Agents Chemother, (2002). , 2727-2734.

[143] Klugman, K. P, & Lonks, J. R. Hidden epidemic of macrolide-resistant pneumococci. Emerg Infect Dis, (2005). , 802-807.

[144] Halpern, M. T, et al. Meta-analysis of bacterial resistance to macrolides. J Antimicrob Chemother, (2005). , 748-757.

Chapter 5

New Frontiers in the Diagnosis and Treatment of Chronic Neutrophilic Lung Diseases

T. Andrew Guess, Amit Gaggar and
Matthew T. Hardison

Additional information is available at the end of the chapter

http://dx.doi.org/10.5772/53834

1. Introduction

Neutrophils, or polymorphonuclear leukocytes (PMNs), are a key component in the innate immune system and a powerful player in host defense. Because of this, PMNs have been studied for over a century, although current understanding of their primary function, trafficking to sites of infection and catabolyzing microbial pathogens, is unchanged. PMNs are viewed by some as mere blunt immune instruments, utilized by the host against a broad array of pathogens. However, a careful review of both neutrophil function and dysfunction reveals a cell of discrete coordination in both normal homeostasis and disease. Herein, we provide a review of neutrophil biology focusing on PMNs role in chronic inflammatory lung disease. We provide a summary of the current knowledge of these cellular first responders and detail novel therapeutics related to combating their dysfunction in chronic disease.

2. Evolutionary origin of neutrophils

The evolutionary origins of the human neutrophil lie in phagocytic cells found in simple organisms. These evolutionary precursors to the human PMNs, originally studied in starfish, were first observed migrating to a site of injury over a century ago. Since the seminal immunological discovery of cells that attack invading pathogens, various phagocytic immune cells along the evolutionary continuum have been described. Phagocytic cells with functions and signaling mechanisms similar to mammalian neutrophils have been described in organisms as simple as the slime mold *Dictyostelium discoideum*. [1] Phagocytes containing bactericidal granules analogous to those in the human neutrophil are found in insects. Although functionally similar, these immune cells differ from their human counterparts significantly in lifespan and nuclear morphology, suggesting that a short-lived, multi-lobed phagocyte is a more recent evolutionary development. [2] This trend continues with non-mammalian vertebrates. Both amphibians and bony fish have granulocytic phagocytes with multi-lobed nuclei that are genetically and morphologically similar to the human PMN. [3] Although the structure, morphology, function, and genetic make-up of neutrophils is highly conserved within mammals, the percentage of total immune cells represented by neutrophils varies significantly. Even within primates neutrophil counts vary a great deal; neutrophils represent approximately 50% of chimpanzee's circulating immune cells, whereas the human neutrophil accounts for almost 70% of white blood cells. [4],[5] The commonality of PMNs and PMN-like cells make it clear that the neutrophil is an ancient player on the immunological stage.

3. Hematopoietic origin, differentiation/maturation of neutrophils

Neutrophil biogenesis occurs in the bone marrow from an undifferentiated hematopoietic stem cell. Regulation of transcription factors through cytokine and growth factor signaling dictates neutrophil differentiation, a process called granulopoiesis. Granulopoiesis is the successive differentiation of a pluripotent hematopoietic stem cell, to a multipotent committed myeloid progenitor cell (myeloblast), to a bipotent granulocyte-macrophage progenitor cell (metamyelocyte) and finally to a unipotent committed granulocyte. The final stage of PMN maturation, or terminal granulopoiesis, is characterized morphologically by the appearance of a multi-lobed granulated nucleus. On a molecular level, granule protein synthesis and granule packaging mark neutrophil maturation. These granules and their cargo proteins are among the primary weapons in neutrophils' antimicrobial arsenal. [6]-[8]Synthesis of granules and granule proteins progresses concurrently with granulopoiesis. Granules are traditionally classified as primary, secondary and tertiary according to the stage of differentiation during which they are formed. This is important because the granules formed at different stages of differentiation exhibit drastically different protein cargo and thus play different roles in the immune and inflammatory response. [9]The array of neutrophilic granule cargo might include myeloperoxidase, lactoferrin, haptoglobin and alpha-1-antitrypsin. [10] Specific granule proteins and their respective roles in neutrophilic lung disease will be addressed below.

4. Release and homeostasis

Once mature, neutrophils are released from the bone marrow. Locally, release of neutrophils into circulation is governed by cytokine signaling. Toll like receptors (TLRs) and granulocyte colony stimulating factor (G-CSF) receptors are crucial in neutrophil production, but CXCR2 and CXCR4 appear to be the primary receptors involved in neutrophil release into the circulation. [11],[12] Whereas activation of CXCR4 favors retention of mature PMNs in the bone marrow, activation of CXCR2 promotes their release into circulation. Under homeostatic conditions a normal human adult produces 1 - 2 X 10[11] neutrophils per day. The rate of neutrophil production and release is dictated largely by G-CSF in a negative feedback mechanism whereby an increasing number of apoptotic neutrophils decreases the amount of G-CSF. The apoptotic neutrophils are phagocytosed by tissue macrophages, which decrease their release of interleukin-23 (IL-23). IL-23 stimulates the release of IL-17 by helper T (T_H) cells. [13] IL-17 is in turn the primary stimulus for the release of G-CSF. Thus, increased controlled destruction of neutrophils leads to decreased levels of macrophage derived IL-23 released by macrophages, IL-17 released by T_H17 cells, G-CSF released by osteoblasts, and thus a decrease in neutrophil synthesis and release. Conversely, IL-17 has been shown to act through p38 MAPK to augment IL-8 release from pulmonary epithelial cells. This mechanism, ideally, allows the body to rapidly speed neutrophil production and release during infection in a regulated fashion to minimize potential damage to the host. [10],[14]Another method by which the host regulates circulating neutrophil numbers is through the phenomenon of margination and demargination. Margination occurs when resting neutrophils travel at a significantly slower pace along the endothelium of the blood vessels. The expression of previously mentioned adhesion molecules creates distinct organ-specific (marginated) pools of cells. Exercise induced stress, infection, or other sources of systemic stress leads to an increase in blood flow, a release of epinephrine and demargination of the neutrophil into the general circulation.[15]

5. Response to infection/smoking

Although the rate of neutrophil production and release may increase during an immunological challenge, as the most populous circulating white blood cells, neutrophils serve as first line responders to injury and infection. During the course of their 6 to 8 hour life span in circulation, neutrophils tend to remain near the vascular endothelium. PMNs constitutively express two glycoprotein ligands, PSGL-1 and L-selectin, allowing neutrophils to detect inflamed or injured endothelium. At sites of inflammation, bacterial peptides such as lipopolysaccharide (LPS), and f-Met-Leu-Phe (fMLP), along with host pro-inflammatory cytokines (i.e., tumor necrosis factor-α [TNF-α]) stimulate the vascular endothelium to produce to adhesion molecules such as lymphocyte function antigen (LFA) and the immunoglobulin-derived intercellular adhesion molecule (ICAM). [4],[15]

The adhesive force between the endothelial adhesion molecules and neutrophil selectins produces a Velcro®-like action that slows the neutrophil down, a process known as rolling. Rolling also prompts the neutrophil to express surface molecules known as β-integrins, which further slow the neutrophil. It is at this early stage that PMNs have already begun to become activated and are preparing the intracellular machinery necessary to combat the invading pathogens. Slow rolling is followed by arrest and firm adhesion via clustering of β2-integrins. Arrest initiates actin polymerization vital to migration across the endothelial surface via a G-protein coupled receptor (GPCR) signaling cascade. [16],[17] Transendothelial migration, or exocytosis, begins as the adhesive force between the neutrophil and endothelium increases and the neutrophil "crawls" in search of a suitable route to cross the vessel wall, either paracellular or transcellular. At this point the neutrophil extends pseudopod-like surface projections that penetrate the endothelium. Upon penetration the neutrophil increases expression of surface integrins and releases proteases that function to break through the vascular basement membrane and into the inflamed tissue. [16]

Once in the interstitium, PMNs must target the specific site of infection amidst large number of healthy cells. This is accomplished by a two pronged method of sensing inflammatory chemoattractant gradients. PMNs sense a chemoattractant gradient of IL-8 produced by damaged host cells and resident monocyte/macrophages through CXCR1 and CXCR2 (both GPCRs), and also detect fMLP (FPR1 receptor) LPS (TLR4), flagellin (TLR5), through pattern recognition receptors. [18] Although PMNs have been traditionally thought to promulgate an active innate immunity with little regulation, more recent evidence suggests that PMNs carefully coordinate a well-tailored immune response. A classic example of this regulated coordination is the elegant response of PMNs to IL-8. [19] As PMNs travel along the IL-8 gradient activation and release of microbicidal molecules occurs in a step-wise manner. With increasing concentrations of IL-8, neutrophils first produce more β-integrins, subsequently begin the oxidative burst, and finally degranulate potent proteases into the intracellular space. [20] The trafficking of neutrophils to sites of inflammation is with dual purpose: 1) to release their antimicrobial arsenal, and 2) to recruit more neutrophils and other innate immune cells to the site of inflammation.

The neutrophil's arsenal includes the following weapons with which the neutrophil attacks pathogens: release of aforementioned granules with their anti-microbial contents, synthesis and release of anti-microbial peptides, production of reactive oxygen species (ROS) during the respiratory/oxidative burst, phagocytosis (mainly utilized to remove debris) and the release of neutrophil extracellular traps (NETs), composed of DNA material that entraps invading pathogens. The second objective is accomplished through the release soluble mediators such as IL-12 and IFN-gamma that form a complex network of recruitment of other neutrophils, dendritic cells, natural killer cells and macrophages. [21] Neutrophils can also act as antigen presenting cells in communication with CD8+ T cells, thus forming a link between innate and adaptive immunity. Such a potent response to injury and inflammation depends on negative feedback mechanisms, the short life span of neutrophils and the clearance of apoptotic neutrophils by macrophages. If left unchecked, the inflammatory response mediated by neutrophils can be a major contributor to chronic disease. [4] (Fig. 1)

Neutrophils are capable of responding to a number of inflammatory stimuli other than infection. Cigarette smoking has been shown to be a primary stimulus for the activation and migration of neutrophils into the tissues. Neutrophil treatment with cigarette smoke induces β_2-integrin activation and firm adhesion to fibrinogen. Increased levels of neutrophil elastase, and matrix metalloproteases has been demonstrated with exposure to cigarette smoke. Furthermore, there is a decrease in superoxide production in the presence of cigarette smoke, indicating that smoking may lead to an impaired response to bacterial challenge.

It is with this potential for destructive dysregulation that we provide the following review of selected neutrophil mediated, inflammatory lung diseases. The definition, etiology, epidemiology, cellular pathophysiology, diagnosis and current treatment of each condition will be discussed briefly. Following each disease will be a discussion of recent advancements in the understanding of the disease and advancements in therapeutics directed toward each condition.

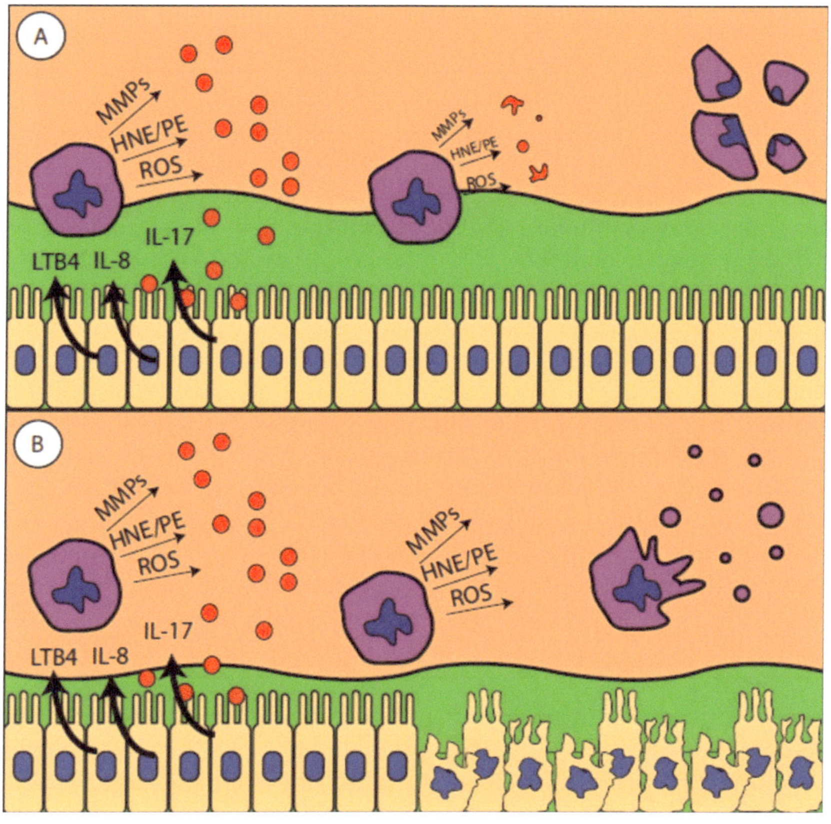

Figure 1. Neutrophils in both normal and chronic inflammatory responses. Neutrophils are recruited into the airway in normal acute information through the release of chemokines such as IL-8, IL-17 and LTB4. Once in the airway they release proteases and reactive oxygen species (ROS) to combat bacteria (shown in red). After the infection in resolved, the neutrophils undergo apoptosis and prevent destructive release of their proteases and ROS into the interstitium. (A) In chronic inflammation, neutrophils continue to release harmful proteases with no pathogen presence. Eventually the neutrophils undergo necrosis which futher damages the epithelium and creates a feed-forward process of disease. (B)

6. COPD

6.1. Overview and epidemiology

Chronic obstructive pulmonary disease (COPD) is marked by progressive and irreversible airway limitation, chronic bronchitis, pulmonary hypertension and emphysema. These tissue changes are secondary to persistent, chronic pulmonary inflammation in response to persistent exposure to toxic gases or particles, primarily tobacco smoke. In addition to a baseline inflammatory state, the disease is associated with frequent exacerbations due to constant inflammation. [22],[23] Although preventable and treatable, COPD is a significant cause of morbidity and mortality worldwide. As the leading cause of pulmonary-related death in the world, COPD was the fifth leading cause of death worldwide in 2001 and is expected to move to third by 2020. [24]

6.2. Etiology

An overwhelming proportion of COPD is related directly to cigarette smoking. Other environmental irritants that have been implicated in the development of COPD include coal and metal mining dust, urban pollution, and indoor cooking with biofuels. [25] Irrespective of secondary irritants, greater than 90% of individuals diagnosed with COPD are current or former smokers. However, only a minority of current and former smokers develop symptomatic COPD (15-20%), suggesting COPD is a confluence of environmental factors and genetic susceptibility. [26] The complex nature of the inflammatory process and its response to environmental factors in COPD confounds the search for individual susceptibility genes. [27] To that end, several genome-wide association studies (GWAS) have been performed with the goal of elucidating the genetic factors related COPD pathogenesis. Unfortunately, even in this current age of rapid whole genome sequencing, multiple GWAS studies have only postulated loose corollaries of genes and association with disease. No genes associated with COPD have displayed a Mendelian mode of inheritance with respect to causation of COPD. [28]

6.3. Pathophysiology

On a cellular level, the pathophysiology of COPD is essentially a heightened, perpetually active inflammatory process. Inflammation is typically localized in the small airways and parenchyma of the lungs, where irritant molecules become trapped. The difference between the normal inflammatory cascade and that seen in COPD is the damage immune cells and their mediators inflict upon the lung tissues due to persistent activation. Lung function decline, characteristic of COPD, is linked to three distinct but synergistic mechanisms: destruction of alveolar walls (emphysema), narrowing of the small airways, and hypersecretion of mucus. [29]

The inflammatory cascade leading to COPD is a complex interaction of immune cells and molecular mediators. The process begins with the inhalation of cigarette smoke or other chemical irritants, which damages the airway epithelium leading to release of chemoattractant molecules. Cigarette smoke was also shown by Braber et al. to induce β2 integrin-dependant migration of neutrophils across endothelial cells. [30] These ligands bind and activate chemokine receptors on circulating neutrophils, helper T cells, cytotoxic T cells and monocytes and recruit them to the lungs. Monocytes migrate across the epithelium and differentiate, joining the resident macrophages. As the congregation of immune cells grows they release proteases, such as matrix metalloproteinase-9 (MMP-9) and human neutrophil elastase (HNE), which degrade connective tissue, particularly elastin, of the alveolar wall, leading to emphysema. [31]-[33] Airway narrowing results from fibroblast proliferation and collagen deposition around the bronchioles in response to TGF B (transforming growth factor) released by macrophages and irritated epithelial cells.

6.4. Role of neutrophils in COPD

Neutrophils themselves are a primary factor in the continuation of the pro-inflammatory state seen in COPD. The hypersecretion of mucus is linked to the accumulation of PMNs. Neutrophil elastase stimulates mucin gene expression; hence goblet cells and mucus glands produce excess mucus, leaving the bronchioles further obstructed. [34],[35] HNE is a one of a family of neutrophil serine proteases that have pluripotent effects in COPD. Not only can HNE degrade the basement membrane but it also directly affects ciliary beat frequency and cleaves CD2, CD4, and CD8 on T-cells, affecting their function. Additionally, HNE cleaves CXCR1 on PMNs, creating an impotent neutrophil that travels to the site of infection but is incapable of acting once it arrives. [36] Furthermore, other neutrophil proteins such as protienase-3, cathepsin G, and myeloperoxidase are all pro-inflammatory molecules released by the neutrophil upon activation or necrosis. [37]

6.5. Diagnosis of COPD

The current standard for COPD diagnosis is spirometry. Lung spirometry measures the volume of exhaled air, thus providing a functional assessment of airway obstruction. Two key spirometric values are FEV1 (forced expiratory volume), the volume of exhaled air over the first second of forced expiration, and FVC (forced vital capacity) or the total volume of air exhaled during forced expiration. These values are interpreted as a ratio (FEV1/FVC) whereby a decreasing value indicates increasing airway obstruction. A ratio less than 0.70 after bronchodilator treatment is diagnostic for COPD. [38],[39] Clinical indications for spirometric evaluation include age greater than 40 years, family history of COPD, past exposure to inhaled irritants, chronic cough and sputum production and dyspnea. [22]

6.6. Traditional COPD therapeutics

Pharmacological therapy of COPD is rooted in combating the symptoms that present secondary to the tissue damage described above. Currently drug therapy is limited to a small cadre of drug classes. Therapeutic agents include bronchodilators, glucocorticosteroids and phosphodiesterase inhibitors. Bronchodilators are the mainstay of COPD therapy. B 2 receptor agonists act on bronchial smooth muscle, promoting relaxation and airway dilation. Both long acting (daily therapy) and short acting (acute exacerbation) formulations are used. [40] Anticholinergics, or acetylcholine antagonists complement the airway dilating mechanism of β-agonists by blocking parasympathetic muscarinic receptors that otherwise cause bronchial smooth muscle contraction. [41] Inhaled glucocorticosteroids aid in controlling inflammation, but are typically only used in conjunction with other drug classes. Oral, or systemic, glucocorticoid therapy is reserved for acute exacerbations because of chronic immunosuppression and undesirable side-effect profiles from long-term daily use. [42]

7. Cystic fibrosis

7.1. Disease overview

Cystic fibrosis (CF) results from a genetic defect in the cystic fibrosis transmembrane conductance regulator (CFTR), an epithelial cell ion transporter. Although the resultant lung pathology is the main source of morbidity and mortality, there is multi-system dysfunction due to the prevalence of the channel in several cell types. The myriad manifestations of CF include lung disease, pancreatic insufficiency (both endocrine and exocrine), male infertility, liver disease, meconium ileus, and distal intestinal obstruction. [43],[44] Among these, the primary cause of morbidity and mortality in cystic fibrosis is pulmonary disease. Pulmonary complications stem from impaired ion transport in the airways, which results in thick mucus, reduced ciliary beat frequency and pathogen clearance from the respiratory tract. These pathogens constantly bombard and eventually colonize the CF patient's airways, which leads to a state of persistent inflammation marked by recurrent infections and exacerbations. [45]

7.2. Epidemiology/prevalence/survival

CF predominately affects Caucasians, and has an estimated prevalence of roughly 80,000 people worldwide. When it was first described in 1938, CF virtually guaranteed death shortly after diagnosis. However, advances in knowledge of the disease process and clinical management of CF have led to improved life expectancy of 25 years in 1985 and currently approaching 40 years. Individuals diagnosed with CF today are expected to survive beyond 50 years of age. [46]

7.3. Etiology

The cystic fibrosis gene is situated on the long arm of chromosome 7. CF mutations are transmitted in an autosomal recessive pattern [47] and over 1500 unique mutations of the CF gene have been identified. [48] Such a large number of different mutations, and the demonstrated influence of other genes (i.e. TGFB1) suggests the probability of considerable variability in genotype, phenotype and disease severity. [49] Indeed, this is the case; symptoms, onset and severity vary widely across the CF population. CF patients are classified I-VI according to the type of defect the mutation causes in the resultant protein. Class I mutations are nonsense or stopgain mutations that cause the protein to be truncated. Class II are typically missense mutations that affect the tertiary structure of the protein and prevent it from trafficking to the cell membrane (this is by far the most common type of mutation seen in CF). The most common of all CFTR mutations is termed ΔF508, a deletion of three nucleotides resulting in a deletion of phenylalanine at position 508, and is a class II mutation. In class III mutations, the CFTR is fully formed and traffics correctly to the cell membrane but does not function properly upon reaching it. Class IV mutations are similar to that of class III but they are solely malfunctions in the opening of the channel. Class V mutations result in less than normal amounts of CFTR, although what is made functions correctly. Finally, class VI mutations are similar to that of class V but they are unique in that what CFTR protein is made is degraded too quickly and there is a functional deficit in the necessary amount of CFTR present on the apical membrane. [50]Typically genotypes in classes I-III have worse phenotypic presentations and higher mortality. Like genotype, sex is also a mortality predictor; males have a higher survival rate than females until the age of 20. [51],[52]

7.4. Pathophysiology

As noted above, CF presents with numerous extra-pulmonary symptoms, but only pulmonary complications will be addressed herein. Pulmonary manifestations of CF can be understood as a stepwise melding of the following pathologic processes:

1. Defective CFTR
2. Reduced ASL height
3. Disrupted mucociliary clearance
4. Colonization/chronic infection/exacerbation
5. Neutrophil dominated inflammation

(1) The underlying genetic defect in CF results in either a dysfunctional or absent CFTR channel. The submucosal glands in the distal airways express CFTR, a protein that spans the membrane of epithelial cells. It employs a cAMP-mediated, PKA activated mechanism to conduct chloride ions across the lipid bilayer. Other functions of CFTR that have been described are affected with varying degrees based on the type of mutation (congenital bilateral absence of the vas deferens). How those secondary functions are altered may explain the phenotypic severity in CF, but dysregulation and dysfunction in chloride conductance is the primary pathology of the CFTR in CF.

(2) Ineffective secretion of chloride anions (and unregulated absorption of sodium ions) leads to a reduced volume of airway surface liquid (ASL) due to the diminished electrolyte content in the airway and very little osmotic pull. In turn, this alters the consistency of airway mucus to a thick, desiccated, hyper-viscous layer that adheres to the airway epithelium. [53]

(3) The adherent mucus creates plaques that obstruct the airways and disrupt the mucociliary clearance mechanism. The detrimental effect of poor mucus clearance is two-fold. First, lung function, as measured by spirometry, declines due to the physical obstruction of the airways. Clogged with mucus plugs, the small airways conduct air less efficiently. Second, the adherent mucus becomes a nidus for infection. [54]

(4) The airways are thus persistently colonized by multiple species of bacteria, namely Pseudamonas aeruginosa, Burkholderia cepacia, Hemophila influezae and Staphylococcus aur-

eus. These organisms are difficult to eradicate in the CF patient, even with continuous prophylactic antibiotic treatment. Colonization is a doorway for infection, and CF is marked by periods of infection and significant decline in lung function known as exacerbations. The etiology of CF exacerbations is closely linked to fluctuations in the balance of bacterial flora in the airway. [55]

(5) Airway obstruction, colonization and episodic exacerbations promote a state of chronic inflammation in CF. In fact, the clinical status of the CF patient, especially during an exacerbation, is tied more closely to the inflammatory response than the quantity and types of organisms responsible for the infection. That inflammatory response is dominated by neutrophils (PMNs) and is responsible for the bulk of tissue damage in the CF airways. Bronchoalveolar lavage and sputum specimens from patients during exacerbation reveal high concentrations of both PMNs and their effectors and signaling molecules, such as neutrophil elastase and IL-8, respectively. [56] IL-8 is a powerful recruiter of PMNs, and excess levels of this signaling molecule likely explains the PMN dominated inflammation in CF. Excess PMN recruitment to the lungs results in the discharge of their destructive weapons (described above) and subsequent killing of pathogens, apoptosis and damage to lung and airway tissue. More often the extreme inflammatory state leads to an aggregation of dying PMNs that result in dysregulated cell lysis, or necrosis, instead of a controlled destruction that mitigates tissue damage. When PMNs undergo necrosis instead of apoptosis they release all of the activated enzymes and molecules designed to destroy pathogen into the interstitial space, further damaging an already taxed pulmonary environment. This damage results in a collection of mucopurulent debris that further clogs airways and provides a breeding ground for further infection. [57]

7.5. Diagnosis of cystic fibrosis

The accepted method for diagnosing CF is by quantitative analysis of the chloride ion content of the sweat. This is based on the premise that the CFTR protein is expressed in sweat glands as well, leading to excessive chloride ion concentration in the sweat. DNA immunoreactive trypsinogen screening techniques are available that detect the presence of many of the common CF mutations. [52],[58] Although not standard, newer diagnostic and screening techniques include genotyping and measurement of the nasal potential difference. No matter what the sweat chloride results, diagnosis of CF remains incomplete without molecular analysis of CFTR gene. Identification of the mutations, and confirmation of their trans state is necessary to provide the patient with an accurate prognosis and clear counseling to parents as to their future reproductive options. Nasal potential difference assesses ion conductance in vivo by observing changes in the voltage potential difference across the nasal epithelium. [59]

7.6. Current cystic fibrosis therapeutics

Advancements in therapeutics in CF in recent decades are the foundation for the prolonged survival of individuals noted above. Unfortunately, almost all current therapies the clinician has at his or her disposal only address the symptoms of CF without correcting the underly-

http://dx.doi.org/10.5772/53834

ing channelopathy. Current CF therapeutics are best understood in relation to how they address the five pathological processes described above. Efforts to address the underlying cause of CF, mutations of the CFTR gene, are underway in the form of gene therapy. The central problem surrounding gene therapy is the search for a suitable delivery mechanism. Viral vectors have been studied, but immune provocation remains to be an obstacle. [60] Reduced ASL height has been successfully addressed with inhaled hypertonic saline and enzymes, such as recombinant human DNAase (dornase alfa). In conjunction with the inhalation therapies noted above, techniques such as breathing exercises, positive expiratory pressure masks, and chest compression (both manual and automated) seek to disrupt the mucus plaques that line the CF airways. Aggressive antibiotic therapy is employed to combat both chronic colonization and acute infections. Although inhaled tobramycin and ciprofloxacin therapy have been effective, the wide array of bacteria in the CF airway precludes development of antibiotic therapy protocol. Finally, high dose ibuprofen and macrolide (typically Azithromycin) treatments stifle the persistent, PMN-dominated inflammation seen in CF. [46],[61],[62] There have been recent exciting discoveries regarding treatment of CF and these will be discussed in a later section.

8. Alpha 1 AT

8.1. Overview/epidemiology

α1-Antitrypsin (A1AT) deficiency (A1AD) is a form of COPD that is an extreme form of the condition, with the potential to develop COPD without excessive smoking. Patients with A1AT deficiency comprise approximately 5% of the global COPD population and have a predicted life span more than 10 years less than those of a life-long smoke with COPD. A1AT is believed by many to be an underreported condition affecting up to 1:2000 people. [63] Although this may seem extremely prevalent, those with the condition only begin to appear symptomatic with cigarette smoking. The underreporting of A1AD may also be due to clinicians giving a diagnosis of idiopathic COPD, or COPD without a known underlying cause. [64]

8.2. Etiology

A1AD is a genetic disorder inherited in an autosomal recessive manner. Patients with A1AT have at least two mutations in a *trans* configuration in the A1AT gene. A1AD patients most often become symptomatic after cigarette smoking, although it is possible to present with emphysema in the third decade of life with no prior tobacco use. Patients present with wheezing, shortness of breath, rales, rhonci, and in some cases, liver failure. [65]

8.3. Pathophysiology

A1AT, an acute phase protein, is member of the serpin family of protease inhibitors. It is produced in the liver and serves to prevent activation and function of the neutrophil serine proteases HNE and proteinase-3. It is normally present at relatively high concentrations (1.5g/L) in the blood and is believed to play a prominent role in resolving inflammation under normal homeostasis. A1AD derived COPD is believed to be due to a protease/antiprotease imbalance in which normal levels of HNE and proteinase-3 (P3) are uninhibited at sites of minor infection or inflammation. [66] The constitutively active HNE and P3 are left unencumbered to degrade extra-cellular matrix and begin a pro-inflammatory cascade of molecules that only further exacerbate the inflammation. Cigarette smoking is so destructive to those with A1AD because cigarette smoke directly inactivates A1AT, wreaking even further havoc on an already taxed system. The pathophysiology of A1AD is similar to that of COPD and thus the underdiagnosis of this condition.

8.4. Role of neutrophils in A1AD

Very similar to the role they play in traditional COPD, PMNs are both effect and maintain inflammation seen in COPD. As producers of HNE they are responsible for the initial pathology seen in the condition. [67]Under normal circumstances, A1AT is loosely bound to HNE, among other serine proteases. However, in the chronic inflammatory condition associated with A1AD, HNE is constantly active and degrades the basement matrix. Furthermore, HNE has been shown to be capable of cleaving the inactive form of MMP-9, pro-MMP-9 to the active form, creating more protease stress on the system. MMP-9 and HNE are capable of degrading multiple matrix proteins present in the lung. This destruction of the basement collagen, elastin, etc. creates a "leaky" vasculature, only making it easier for other immune cells to move into the lung interstitium. [68] This movement of cells and proteins into the intracellular space brings with it fluid from the circulation and edema results. As the producers of HNE, neutrophils are integral to the pathogenesis and continuation of A1AD associated COPD.

8.5. Diagnosis of A1AD

Diagnosis of A1AD is only made in those cases of COPD where there is an unexplained cause of the condition. A1AT serum levels are measured using enzyme linked adsorbent assays (ELISA), or more recently mass spectrometry. Like CF, there is a spectrum of phenotypes that are observed in the condition and they are categorized based upon the circulating levels of A1AT. Patients with the most severe phenotype are those individuals with concentrations less than 15% of normal in their serum. [69]

8.6. Treatment of A1AD

Because of the nature of the disease treatment of A1AD is very similar to that of traditional COPD, with one exception. Patients with a severe lung phenotype are treated with intravenous infusion of A1AT isolated from human serum. [70] Additionally, liver transplant has been utilized to address the absence of circulating A1AT. [71] In addition to these therapies, the common treatments for COPD mentioned previously are employed to address the specific symptoms of A1AD.

http://dx.doi.org/10.5772/53834

9. Neutrophilic/steroid resistant asthma

9.1. Overview/epidemiology

Asthma was first defined in 1860 by Salter, a British clinician who ascertained that attacks were related to smooth muscle contraction. Asthma, at its core, is a chronic airway disease characterized by wheezing, coughing, and breathlessness with variable airway obstruction on pulmonary function testing. Asthma is a relatively common disease; recent reports by the Center for Disease Control (CDC) place its prevalence at approximately 12% (children) and 10% (adults) in the US. (www.cdc.gov) There appears to be a predominance of childhood asthma in non-Hispanic blacks, whereas non-Hispanic Whites, Hispanics, Asians, and Native Americans all have similar frequencies of asthma. Additionally, the condition is significantly more common among females than males.

9.2. Etiology

The development of asthma is thought to be associated with three major risk factors: genetic predisposition, and occupational and environmental factors. Although a precise list of genes associated with the atopic response in human has yet to be collated, GWAS studies in human, and canines have revealed multiple loci related to the IgE response known to be important in the etiology of asthma. [72],[73]

9.3. Pathophysiology

Asthma begins in the airways with host contact of an allergen, following this, specific IGE antibodies are upregulated and initiate mast cell activation. Mast cell activation, in turn begins the early and late phase response. The early phase response is mediated by histamine, leukotriene C4, D4, and E4, and prostoglandin D2. After the early phase/hypersensitivity response, that late phase response begins. Eosinophils, basophils, neutrophils, and T cells are all recruited to the airway and produce inflammatory cytokines that propogate the allergic response that is a hallmark of asthma.

9.4. Role of neutrophils in neutrophilic and steroid-resistant asthma

Asthma is typically thought of as an eosinophilic disease, yet there have been numerous studies reporting an increase in neutrophil number and activation in sputum collected from steroid-resistant asthma patients. There are reports of up to 50% of asthma cases that have an increase in IL-8 and neutrophil burden, separate from eosinophilic inflammation. [74],[75] Because of the variability seen in primary immune cell burden in asthma neutrophilic asthma has recently begun to be viewed as a specific sub-type of the condition. [76] Patients with neutrophilic asthma have a more severe progression of disease, respond poorly to therapy, and are burdened with much high health care costs than typical asthma patients. Unfortunately, there is little, if any, established dogma regarding neutrophilic asthma. Studies have only been able to describe correlative relationships between neutrophil burden and the phenotypic profile observed in neutrophilic asthma patients. [77] There has been extensive work performed investigating the role of MMP-9 in the pathogenesis of asthma. In a report by Cundall et al the authors state that MMP-9 concentrations in BAL fluid correlate with eosinophils but not neutrophil or monocyte/macrophage counts. [78] They hypothesize that PMNs and macrophages release MMP-9 which breaks down the basement membrane, making it easier for the eosinophils to migrate into the airways. In another study, MMP-9 levels in BAL fluid were correlated significantly with decreases in FEV1 seen in asthma patients.

HNE, another potent neutrophil derived protease, has also been correlated with symptoms of asthma. [79] Patients with allergic rhinitis has significantly elevated levels of HNE in their nasal lavage compared to control patients in which no rhinitis was observed. To add to the myriad of evidence that neutrophils are at the very least, associated with asthma, a study by Norzila et al demonstrated that myeloperoxidase (MPO), a neutrophil mediator of the oxidative burst, is elevated in induced sputum collected from certain asthma patients compared to control patients. [80] Because MPO, HNE, and MMP-9 are all contained in intracellular granules of the neutrophil it is evidence that neutrophils present in/around the lung in asthma patients are activated and degranulate.

9.5. Diagnosis of asthma

Diagnosis of asthma is made through evaluation of symptoms and pulmonary function testing (PFT) via spirometry. An increase in FEV of ≥15% in conjunction with reported wheezing, chest tightness, and coughing is diagnostic for asthma. A difficulty arises when patients present with normal spirometry results. To address this, home PFT devices are available to record lung function data over a period of time to encapsulate more data points. Additionally, controlled exacerbation of asthma attacks with methacholine in the clinician's office is a reliable method of eliciting the necessary response to confirm a diagnosis of asthma. [81]

9.6. Traditional asthma therapeutics

Similar to the other lung diseases discussed in this chapter, treatment of asthma is relegated to management of symptoms. Monitoring of frequency and severity of attacks is vital to administering correct dosages of medication. Patients are encouraged to keep records of attacks with information regarding date/time, location, duration, and triggers. The standard treatment of asthma is glucocorticoid (GC) inhaler with a long-acting β-agonist. [82] The GC treatment is directed at reducing the constant inflammatory state, whereas the β-agonist is a bronchodilator intended to ameliorate airway obstruction. So physicians will also prescribe the use of IgE inhibitors or neutralizing antibodies such as omaluzimab to combat the high levels of the pro-inflammatory molecule. [83] In neutrophil associated and steroid-resistant asthma, clinicians have fewer options with which to treat this potentially deadly condition. A patient's response to a two week trial of traditional asthma therapy will indicate whether or not they are a candidate for alternative asthma therapy. Because certain forms of asthma are refractory to GC therapy, the focus of treatment in such patients shifts to a more aggressive immunosuppressive approach. Treatment with cyclosporine, tacrolimus, and methotrexate have been associated with some benefit, although the risk of side effects is significantly higher in these classes of medicines. Finally, IV immunoglobulin therapy is utilized in extreme cases, but due to its expense and limited evidence of efficacy, its use is not widespread. Because of the lack of knowledge about the cellular and molecular etiology of neutrophilic asthma, current therapies are limited to those already employed in traditional asthma. As might be expected, these have limited efficacy in patients diagnosed with neutrophilic asthma.

10. Novel therapeutics in neutrophilic lung diseases

With better understanding of neutrophilic lung disease has come more advanced and targeted therapeutics. Towards that end, recent work by the Blalock and Gaggar groups at the University of Alabama at Birmingham (UAB) has expanded the role of PMNs in multiple chronic inflammatory lung diseases, including COPD, CF, and BOS. They described a novel concept of neutrophils proteases producing a neutrophil chemokine from extra-cellular collagen that acted in a feed-forward mechanism of disease. Seminal papers by Weathington et al and Gaggar et al detail the step-wise manner in which IL-8 draws PMNs into the interstitium, upon activation they release MMP-8 and MMP-9 which perform an initial digestion of collagen from macromolecule size. Subsequently, neutrophils release prolyl endopeptidase (PE), a serine protease previously only known to be a processor of neuropeptides. PE performs the final digestion of collagen to the tri-peptide proline-glycine-proline (PGP) from the PPGP amino acid motif that is repeated over 40 times throughout a single collagen molecule. [84],[85] PGP binds to the same receptors as IL-8, CXCR1 and CXCR2 acting a neutrophil chemoattractant and activator. [86] The authors showed that not only are the proteases responsible for PGP production present and elevated in BAL fluid collected from COPD and CF patients, both stable and in exacerbations, but PGP is also measurably elevated by mass spectrometry in the BAL fluid of such patients and correlates with PMN burden in disease. [39],[87],[88] These data indicate that not only is PGP a potential biomarker for chronic inflammatory neutrophilic lung disease, but the system of proteases responsible for PGP's production, and the receptors upon which it acts are potential targets for the development of novel precise therapeutics. Furthermore, work by Hardison et al, and Braber et al have demonstrated that cigarette smoke and its constituents are capable of acetylating PGP into the more potent and stable n-terminal acetylated form, AcPGP. [89],[90] AcPGP has proven to be resistant to degradation by leukotriene A4 hydrolase (LTA4H), a hydrolase/amino-peptidase also produced a number of cells, including neutrophils. In a 2010 Science paper, Snelgrove et al described a novel function for the dual purpose enzyme in resolving acute neutrophilic inflammation in a mouse model of influenza. [91] It would be extremely useful to have pharmaco-interventions able to modulate the PGP system of neutrophil inflammation, either at the genesis (MMP, PE) or terminus (CXCR, LTA4H).

Although any therapeutics derived from such work may be years away from fruition, there are other recent advancements that are already making an impact on patient morbidity and mortality. Kalydeco, a drug produced by Vertex Pharmaceuticals is the first drug developed that addresses the underlying genetic cause of CF. First released on the market in January of 2012, it is effective in patients that carry the G115D amino acid change. [92] This is a class III mutation in which the protein traffics the cell surface but the channel does not function properly. Kalydeco interacts with the channel and increases the open probability of the channel. Another Vertex product, currently titled VX-809, is designed to act in patients with class II mutations (i.e., ΔF508). VX-809 acts in the endoplasmic reticulum, allowing improperly folded CF protein to pool and undergo corrected folding which results in trafficking to the cell membrane. [93] Both Vertex products are the result of so-called high throughput small molecule screening in which hundreds of thousands of small molecules are screened in a recombinant cell-based assay for an effect on cell function. The discovery of drugs that address the underlying genetics cause is an exciting advancement in any genetic disease, but made even more so by the fact that CF is one of the more common, and fatal diseases caused by a genetic malformation. Whether any of these drugs change the number or activation state of PMNs in the airway is currently unknown

Patients with COPD, an even larger cohort than those with CF may also soon benefit from new therapies targeted at resolving the underlying cause rather than merely treating symptoms. There is currently only a single phosphodiesterase 4 (PDE4) inhibitor, Daliresp that is approved for treatment of COPD in the United States. However, there are clinical trials currently underway researching the effects of multiple other PDE4 inhibitors. [94] PD4 is a cAMP specific phosphodiesterase present, primarily, in inflammatory cells and also in epithelial cells. Treatment with Daliresp has been shown to reduce the release of pro-inflammatory cytokines by neutrophils and resident monocyte/macrophages. Unfortunately, there are several side effects associated with Daliresp and thus the need for better, more targeted PDE4 inhibitors is apparent. Additionally, there have been recent advancements made in traditional COPD therapies. The development of ultra-long acting β2 agonists has proved beneficial in a number of lung diseases, including COPD, A1AT, and asthma. [95] Research is also underway into the identification of biomarkers for smokers who will develop COPD, allowing treatment or prevention to possibly begin earlier. Investigators at Weill Cornell College of Medicine are using a metabolomics approach in a cohort of smokers to establish a thorough catalogue of abnormal cell changes in airway epithelium after cigarette smoking. (weill.cornell.edu) Utilizing serum, epithelial lining fluid, and airway epithelial samples, Dr. Crystal's group aims to identify the early changes in airway epithelium that indicate if a patient will develop COPD later.

McNab et al recently published work detailing their investigation of "compound cg," a small molecule that assists in reducing aggregates of abnormal A1AT protein. [96] GC was effective in an *in vitro* model of A1AT deficiency and showed significant reduction in At1AT aggregates by both immunohistochemistry and Western blot analysis. Gene therapy is another approach, also applicable to CF that is being investigated as a potential source of curing the disease in A1AT deficiency. A group at UMass has pioneered a dual gene therapy approach that addressed both the lung malfunction and liver disease so often associated with aggregation of mutant protein. In utilizing an adeno-associated virus (AAV) to introduce corrected protein product in the lung, and microRNAs (miRNA) in the liver to reduce production of dysfunctional protein, the investigators have presented the possibility of curative therapy for patients with A1AT deficiency. [97]

http://dx.doi.org/10.5772/53834

Many of the therapies previously mentioned are also in use in the treatment of PMN-related or glucocorticoid resistant asthma. The PDE4 inhibitors, along with ultra-long acting β2 agonists have begun to be used in combating the airway dysfunction associated with asthma. [98] There is work being done to abrogate the ability of inflammatory cells such as neutrophils to bind adhesion molecules such as the integrin VLA-4. [99] Furthermore, kinase inhibitors being investigated that target p38 MAPK and PI3K would also effect neutrophil recruitment and activation in asthma. [100]

11. Conclusion

Chronic neutrophilic airway inflammation is a clinically similar, but foundationally heterogeneous cohort of disease. Although neutrophils are necessary and effective components of the innate immune system in resolving infection, when dysregulated, they can be potent mediators of devastating inflammation. Current therapeutics in a variety of neutrophilic lung diseases fail to address the underlying causes of the conditions and yield questionable benefit to patients. Fortunately, advances in identifications of biomarkers such as PGP and others afford the opportunity to develop targeted therapeutics aimed at resolving and preventing the progressive destruction that is a hallmark of chronic neutrophilic lung disease.

Author details

T. Andrew Guess[1], Amit Gaggar[2] and Matthew T. Hardison[3*]

*Address all correspondence to: mthardis@bcmedu

1 University of Alabama at Birmingham Medical School, Birmingham, AL, USA

2 Division of Pulmonary, Allergy, and Critical Care Medicine, Department of Medicine, University of Alabama at Birmingham, Birmingham, AL, USA

3 Department of Molecular and Human Genetics, Baylor College of Medicine, Houston, TX, USA

References

[1] Chen, G., Zhuchenko, O. & Kuspa, A. Immune-like phagocyte activity in the social amoeba. *Science* 317, 678-681 (2007).

[2] Ribeiro, C. & Brehelin, M. Insect haemocytes: what type of cell is that? *J Insect Physiol* 52, 417-429 (2006).

[3] Robert, J. & Ohta, Y. Comparative and developmental study of the immune system in Xenopus. *Dev Dyn* 238, 1249-1270 (2009).

[4] Amulic, B., Cazalet, C., Hayes, G.L., Metzler, K.D., Zychlinsky, A. Neutrophil Function: From Mechanisms to Disease. *Annual Review of Immunology* 30, 30 (2012).

[5] Ihrig, M., Tassinary, L.G., Bernacky, B. & Keeling, M.E. Hematologic and serum biochemical reference intervals for the chimpanzee (Pan troglodytes) categorized by age and sex. *Comp Med* 51, 30-37 (2001).

[6] Mora-Jensen, H., *et al.* Technical advance: immunophenotypical characterization of human neutrophil differentiation. *J Leukoc Biol* 90, 629-634.

[7] Theilgaard-Monch, K., *et al.* The transcriptional program of terminal granulocytic differentiation. *Blood* 105, 1785-1796 (2005).

[8] Theilgaard-Monch, K., Porse, B.T. & Borregaard, N. Systems biology of neutrophil differentiation and immune response. *Curr Opin Immunol* 18, 54-60 (2006).

[9] Le Cabec, V., Cowland, J.B., Calafat, J. & Borregaard, N. Targeting of proteins to granule subsets is determined by timing and not by sorting: The specific granule protein NGAL is localized to azurophil granules when expressed in HL-60 cells. *Proc Natl Acad Sci U S A* 93, 6454-6457 (1996).

[10] Borregaard, N. Neutrophils, from marrow to microbes. *Immunity* 33, 657-670.

[11] Gladigau, G., *et al.* A role for toll-like receptor mediated signals in neutrophils in the pathogenesis of the anti-phospholipid syndrome. *PLoS One* 7, e42176.

[12] Eash, K.J., Greenbaum, A.M., Gopalan, P.K. & Link, D.C. CXCR2 and CXCR4 antagonistically regulate neutrophil trafficking from murine bone marrow. *J Clin Invest* 120, 2423-2431.

[13] Dubin, P.J., *et al.* Interleukin-23-mediated inflammation in Pseudomonas aeruginosa pulmonary infection. *Infect Immun* 80, 398-409.

[14] Linden, A., Laan, M. & Anderson, G.P. Neutrophils, interleukin-17A and lung disease. *Eur Respir J* 25, 159-172 (2005).

[15] Finn, A., Strobel, S., Levin, M. & Klein, N. Endotoxin-induced neutrophil adherence to endothelium: relationship to CD11b/CD18 and L-selectin expression and matrix disruption. *Ann N Y Acad Sci* 725, 173-182 (1994).

[16] Ley, K., Laudanna, C., Cybulsky, M.I. & Nourshargh, S. Getting to the site of inflammation: the leukocyte adhesion cascade updated. *Nat Rev Immunol* 7, 678-689 (2007).

[17] Zarbock, A. & Ley, K. Mechanisms and consequences of neutrophil interaction with the endothelium. *Am J Pathol* 172, 1-7 (2008).

[18] Bellocchio, S., *et al.* TLRs govern neutrophil activity in aspergillosis. *J Immunol* 173, 7406-7415 (2004).

[19] Burg, N.D. & Pillinger, M.H. The neutrophil: function and regulation in innate and humoral immunity. *Clin Immunol* 99, 7-17 (2001).

[20] Malerba, M., *et al.* Neutrophilic inflammation and IL-8 levels in induced sputum of alpha-1-antitrypsin PiMZ subjects. *Thorax* 61, 129-133 (2006).

[21] Nathan, C. Neutrophils and immunity: challenges and opportunities. *Nat Rev Immunol* 6, 173-182 (2006).

[22] Disease, G.I.f.C.O.L. Pocket Guide to COPD Diagnosis, Management, and Prevention. (2011).

[23] Hogg, J.C. & Timens, W. The pathology of chronic obstructive pulmonary disease. *Annu Rev Pathol* 4, 435-459 (2009).

[24] Buist, A.S., *et al.* International variation in the prevalence of COPD (the BOLD Study): a population-based prevalence study. *Lancet* 370, 741-750 (2007).

[25] Lomas, D.A. & Silverman, E.K. The genetics of chronic obstructive pulmonary disease. *Respir Res* 2, 20-26 (2001).

[26] Cox, L.A., Jr. A mathematical model of protease-antiprotease homeostasis failure in chronic obstructive pulmonary disease (COPD). *Risk Anal* 29, 576-586 (2009).

[27] Barnes, P.J. Genetics and pulmonary medicine. 9. Molecular genetics of chronic obstructive pulmonary disease. *Thorax* 54, 245-252 (1999).

[28] Pillai, S.G., *et al.* A genome-wide association study in chronic obstructive pulmonary disease (COPD): identification of two major susceptibility loci. *PLoS Genet* 5, e1000421 (2009).

[29] Barnes, P.J., Shapiro, S.D. & Pauwels, R.A. Chronic obstructive pulmonary disease: molecular and cellular mechanisms. *Eur Respir J* 22, 672-688 (2003).

[30] Braber, S., *et al.* Cigarette smoke-induced lung emphysema in mice is associated with prolyl endopeptidase, an enzyme involved in collagen breakdown. *Am J Physiol Lung Cell Mol Physiol* 300, L255-265 (2011).

[31] Chakrabarti, S. & Patel, K.D. Regulation of matrix metalloproteinase-9 release from IL-8-stimulated human neutrophils. *J Leukoc Biol* 78, 279-288 (2005).

[32] Chakrabarti, S., Zee, J.M. & Patel, K.D. Regulation of matrix metalloproteinase-9 (MMP-9) in TNF-stimulated neutrophils: novel pathways for tertiary granule release. *J Leukoc Biol* 79, 214-222 (2006).

[33] Geraghty, P., *et al.* Neutrophil elastase up-regulates cathepsin B and matrix metalloprotease-2 expression. *J Immunol* 178, 5871-5878 (2007).

[34] Barnes, P.J. Immunology of asthma and chronic obstructive pulmonary disease. *Nat Rev Immunol* 8, 183-192 (2008).

[35] Caramori, G., *et al.* Mucin expression in peripheral airways of patients with chronic obstructive pulmonary disease. *Histopathology* 45, 477-484 (2004).

[36] Hartl, D., *et al.* Cleavage of CXCR1 on neutrophils disables bacterial killing in cystic fibrosis lung disease. *Nat Med* 13, 1423-1430 (2007).

[37] Hardison, M.T., Jackson, P.L., Blalock, J.E., Gaggar, A. Protease release from neutrophils in inflammation: impact on innate immunity seen in chronic pulmonary disease. in *Handbook of Granulocytes: Classification, Toxic Materials Produced and Pathology* (ed. Haag, R.) 249-270 (Nova Bioscience, 2009).

[38] O'Reilly, P., *et al.* N-alpha-PGP and PGP, potential biomarkers and therapeutic targets for COPD. *Respir Res* 10, 38 (2009).

[39] Djekic, U.V., Gaggar, A. & Weathington, N.M. Attacking the multi-tiered proteolytic pathology of COPD: new insights from basic and translational studies. *Pharmacol Ther* 121, 132-146 (2009).

[40] Sutherland, E.R. & Cherniack, R.M. Management of chronic obstructive pulmonary disease. *N Engl J Med* 350, 2689-2697 (2004).

[41] Cazzola, M., Page, C.P., Calzetta, L. & Matera, M.G. Pharmacology and therapeutics of bronchodilators. *Pharmacol Rev* 64, 450-504.

[42] Restrepo, R.D. A stepwise approach to management of stable COPD with inhaled pharmacotherapy: a review. *Respir Care* 54, 1058-1081 (2009).

[43] Borowitz, D., *et al.* Gastrointestinal outcomes and confounders in cystic fibrosis. *J Pediatr Gastroenterol Nutr* 41, 273-285 (2005).

[44] Hodges, C.A., Palmert, M.R. & Drumm, M.L. Infertility in females with cystic fibrosis is multifactorial: evidence from mouse models. *Endocrinology* 149, 2790-2797 (2008).

[45] Lobo, J., Rojas-Balcazar, J.M. & Noone, P.G. Recent advances in cystic fibrosis. *Clin Chest Med* 33, 307-328.

[46] Cohen-Cymberknoh, M., Shoseyov, D. & Kerem, E. Managing cystic fibrosis: strategies that increase life expectancy and improve quality of life. *Am J Respir Crit Care Med* 183, 1463-1471.

[47] Kerem, E., *et al.* Clinical and genetic comparisons of patients with cystic fibrosis, with or without meconium ileus. *J Pediatr* 114, 767-773 (1989).

[48] Strausbaugh, S.D. & Davis, P.B. Cystic fibrosis: a review of epidemiology and pathobiology. *Clin Chest Med* 28, 279-288 (2007).

[49] Drumm, M.L., *et al.* Genetic modifiers of lung disease in cystic fibrosis. *N Engl J Med* 353, 1443-1453 (2005).

[50] Hull, J. Cystic fibrosis transmembrane conductance regulator dysfunction and its treatment. *J R Soc Med* 105 Suppl 2, S2-8.

[51] Fass, P.S. & Degler, C.N. Of genes and men. *Rev Am Hist* 20, 235-241 (1992).

[52] Lai, H.J., Cheng, Y., Cho, H., Kosorok, M.R. & Farrell, P.M. Association between initial disease presentation, lung disease outcomes, and survival in patients with cystic fibrosis. *Am J Epidemiol* 159, 537-546 (2004).

[53] Rowe, S.M., Miller, S. & Sorscher, E.J. Cystic fibrosis. *N Engl J Med* 352, 1992-2001 (2005).

[54] Rowe, S.M. & Clancy, J.P. Advances in cystic fibrosis therapies. *Curr Opin Pediatr* 18, 604-613 (2006).

[55] Goss, C.H. & Burns, J.L. Exacerbations in cystic fibrosis. 1: Epidemiology and pathogenesis. *Thorax* 62, 360-367 (2007).

[56] Witko-Sarsat, V., Sermet-Gaudelus, I., Lenoir, G. & Descamps-Latscha, B. Inflammation and CFTR: might neutrophils be the key in cystic fibrosis? *Mediators Inflamm* 8, 7-11 (1999).

[57] Koehler, D.R., Downey, G.P., Sweezey, N.B., Tanswell, A.K. & Hu, J. Lung inflammation as a therapeutic target in cystic fibrosis. *Am J Respir Cell Mol Biol* 31, 377-381 (2004).

[58] Laguna, T.A., *et al.* Comparison of quantitative sweat chloride methods after positive newborn screen for cystic fibrosis. *Pediatr Pulmonol* 47, 736-742 (2011).

[59] Flume, P.A. & Stenbit, A. Making the diagnosis of cystic fibrosis. *Am J Med Sci* 335, 51-54 (2008).

[60] Griesenbach, U. & Alton, E.W. Current status and future directions of gene and cell therapy for cystic fibrosis. *BioDrugs* 25, 77-88.

[61] Flume, P.A., *et al.* Cystic fibrosis pulmonary guidelines: treatment of pulmonary exacerbations. *Am J Respir Crit Care Med* 180, 802-808 (2009).

[62] Flume, P.A., *et al.* Cystic fibrosis pulmonary guidelines: airway clearance therapies. *Respir Care* 54, 522-537 (2009).

[63] Kauppi, P. & Jokelainen, K. [Alpha-1 antitrypsin deficiency]. *Duodecim* 127, 1911-1918.

[64] Clancy, J. & Nobes, M. Chronic obstructive pulmonary disease: nature-nurture interactions. *Br J Nurs* 21, 772-781.

[65] Stoller, J.K. & Aboussouan, L.S. A review of alpha1-antitrypsin deficiency. *Am J Respir Crit Care Med* 185, 246-259.

[66] Greene, C.M., Hassan, T., Molloy, K. & McElvaney, N.G. The role of proteases, endoplasmic reticulum stress and SERPINA1 heterozygosity in lung disease and alpha-1 anti-trypsin deficiency. *Expert Rev Respir Med* 5, 395-411.

[67] Clemmensen, S.N., *et al.* Alpha-1-antitrypsin is produced by human neutrophil granulocytes and their precursors and liberated during granule exocytosis. *Eur J Haematol* 86, 517-530.

[68] Bergin, D.A., *et al.* alpha-1 Antitrypsin regulates human neutrophil chemotaxis induced by soluble immune complexes and IL-8. *J Clin Invest* 120, 4236-4250.

[69] Campos, M., Shmuels, D. & Walsh, J. Detection of alpha-1 antitrypsin deficiency in the US. *Am J Med* 125, 623-624.

[70] Mohanka, M., Khemasuwan, D. & Stoller, J.K. A review of augmentation therapy for alpha-1 antitrypsin deficiency. *Expert Opin Biol Ther* 12, 685-700.

[71] Lee, S.M., Speeg, K.V., Pollack, M.S. & Sharkey, F.E. Progression of morphological changes after transplantation of a liver with heterozygous alpha-1 antitrypsin deficiency. *Hum Pathol* 43, 753-756.

[72] Barnes, K.C. Successfully mapping novel asthma loci by GWAS. *Lancet* 378, 967-968.

[73] Hirota, T., *et al.* Genome-wide association study identifies three new susceptibility loci for adult asthma in the Japanese population. *Nat Genet* 43, 893-896.

[74] Bousquet, J., *et al.* Eosinophilic inflammation in asthma. *N Engl J Med* 323, 1033-1039 (1990).

[75] Fahy, J.V., Kim, K.W., Liu, J. & Boushey, H.A. Prominent neutrophilic inflammation in sputum from subjects with asthma exacerbation. *J Allergy Clin Immunol* 95, 843-852 (1995).

[76] Douwes, J., Gibson, P., Pekkanen, J. & Pearce, N. Non-eosinophilic asthma: importance and possible mechanisms. *Thorax* 57, 643-648 (2002).

[77] Kamath, A.V., Pavord, I. D., Ruparelia, P. R., Chilvers, E. R. Is the neutrophil the key effector cell in severe asthma? *Thorax* 60, 2 (2005).

[78] Cundall, M., *et al.* Neutrophil-derived matrix metalloproteinase-9 is increased in severe asthma and poorly inhibited by glucocorticoids. *J Allergy Clin Immunol* 112, 1064-1071 (2003).

[79] Baines, K.J., Simpson, J.L., Wood, L.G., Scott, R.J. & Gibson, P.G. Systemic upregulation of neutrophil alpha-defensins and serine proteases in neutrophilic asthma. *Thorax* 66, 942-947 (2011).

[80] Norzila, M.Z., Fakes, K., Henry, R.L., Simpson, J. & Gibson, P.G. Interleukin-8 secretion and neutrophil recruitment accompanies induced sputum eosinophil activation in children with acute asthma. *Am J Respir Crit Care Med* 161, 769-774 (2000).

[81] Nair, P., Dasgupta, A., Brightling, C.E. & Chung, K.F. How to diagnose and phenotype asthma. *Clin Chest Med* 33, 445-457 (2012).

[82] Spangler, D.L. The role of inhaled corticosteroids in asthma treatment: a health economic perspective. *Am J Manag Care* 18, S35-39 (2012).

[83] Barnes, P.J., Nicolini, G., Bizzi, A., Spinola, M. & Singh, D. Do inhaled corticosteroid/long-acting beta2-agonist fixed combinations provide superior clinical benefits compared with separate inhalers? A literature reappraisal. *Allergy Asthma Proc* 33, 140-144 (2012).

[84] Gaggar, A., *et al.* A novel proteolytic cascade generates an extracellular matrix-derived chemoattractant in chronic neutrophilic inflammation. *J Immunol* 180, 5662-5669 (2008).

[85] Weathington, N.M., *et al.* A novel peptide CXCR ligand derived from extracellular matrix degradation during airway inflammation. *Nat Med* 12, 317-323 (2006).

[86] Hardison, M.T., *et al.* The presence of a matrix-derived neutrophil chemoattractant in bronchiolitis obliterans syndrome after lung transplantation. *J Immunol* 182, 4423-4431 (2009).

[87] Gaggar, A., *et al.* Matrix metalloprotease-9 dysregulation in lower airway secretions of cystic fibrosis patients. *Am J Physiol Lung Cell Mol Physiol* 293, L96-L104 (2007).

[88] Gaggar, A., Rowe, S.M., Matthew, H. & Blalock, J.E. Proline-Glycine-Proline (PGP) and High Mobility Group Box Protein-1 (HMGB1): Potential Mediators of Cystic Fibrosis Airway Inflammation. *Open Respir Med J* 4, 32-38.

[89] Hardison, M.T., Brown, M.D., Snelgrove, R.J., Blalock, J.E. & Jackson, P. Cigarette smoke enhances chemotaxis via acetylation of proline-glycine-proline. *Front Biosci (Elite Ed)* 4, 2402-2409 (2011).

[90] Braber, S., *et al.* Cigarette smoke-induced lung emphysema in mice is associated with prolyl endopeptidase, an enzyme involved in collagen breakdown. *Am J Physiol Lung Cell Mol Physiol* (2011).

[91] Snelgrove, R.J., *et al.* A critical role for LTA4H in limiting chronic pulmonary neutrophilic inflammation. *Science* 330, 90-94 (2010).

[92] Hull, J. Cystic fibrosis transmembrane conductance regulator dysfunction and its treatment. *J R Soc Med* 105 Suppl 2, S2-8 (2012).

[93] Kim Chiaw, P., Eckford, P.D. & Bear, C.E. Insights into the mechanisms underlying CFTR channel activity, the molecular basis for cystic fibrosis and strategies for therapy. *Essays Biochem* 50, 233-248 (2011).

[94] Michalski, J.M., Golden, G., Ikari, J. & Rennard, S.I. PDE4: a novel target in the treatment of chronic obstructive pulmonary disease. *Clin Pharmacol Ther* 91, 134-142 (2012).

[95] Vogelmeier, C., Magnussen, H., LaForce, C., Owen, R. & Kramer, B. Profiling the bronchodilator effects of the novel ultra-long-acting beta2-agonist indacaterol against established treatments in chronic obstructive pulmonary disease. *Ther Adv Respir Dis* 5, 345-357 (2012).

[96] McNab, G.L., Dafforn, T.R., Wood, A., Sapey, E. & Stockley, R.A. A novel model and molecular therapy for Z alpha-1 antitrypsin deficiency. *Mamm Genome* 23, 241-249 (2012).

[97] Flotte, T.R. & Mueller, C. Gene therapy for alpha-1 antitrypsin deficiency. *Hum Mol Genet* 20, R87-92 (2011).

[98] Varsano, S. [Perspectives in future asthma therapy]. *Harefuah* 151, 225-229, 253 (2012).

[99] Singh, J., *et al.* Rational design of potent and selective VLA-4 inhibitors and their utility in the treatment of asthma. *Curr Top Med Chem* 4, 1497-1507 (2004).

[100] Mercado, N., *et al.* p38 mitogen-activated protein kinase-gamma inhibition by long-acting beta2 adrenergic agonists reversed steroid insensitivity in severe asthma. *Mol Pharmacol* 80, 1128-1135 (2011).

Chapter 6

Expiratory Flow Limitation in Intra and Extrathoracic Respiratory Disorders: Use of the Negative Expiratory Pressure Technique – Review and Recent Developments

Ahmet Baydur

Additional information is available at the end of the chapter

http://dx.doi.org/10.5772/53270

1. Introduction

1.1. Definition

Expiratory flow limitation (EFL) is defined as an absence in increase in flow with application of negative expiratory pressure (NEP) during quiet breathing (Koulouris et al., 1994). The test is a simple, noninvasive, practical and accurate technique.

Application of the NEP technique provides a simple, rapid, non-invasive, and reliable test to detect tidal expiratory flow limitation; b) it does not require a body-box or cooperation on the patient's part; c) it can be applied in any posture, during mechanical ventilation, and during exercise; d) it provides new insights into the physiology and pathophysiology of several diseases and the symptom of dyspnea.

2. Negative expiratory pressure technique (NEP) – Methodology

In the last 2 decades, expiratory flow limitation (EFL) in patients with various respiratory disorders has been studied extensively using the negative expiratory pressure technique (NEP). This method does not require performance of forced expiratory maneuvers or the body plethysmograph (D'Angelo et al., 1993; Koulouris et al., 1995; Valta et al., 1994). It consists of applying a small negative pressure (3–10 cm H_2O, depending on the circumstances) at the onset of tidal expiration and comparing the ensuing expiration flow-volume curve with that of the preceding control expiration (Figures 1-3).

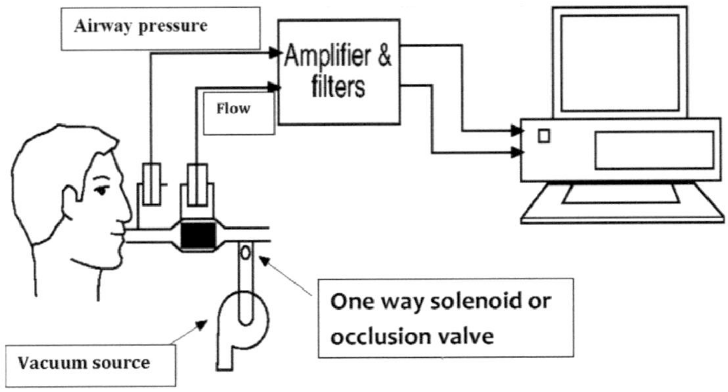

Figure 1. Schema of negative expiratory pressure (NEP) setup to assess expiratory flow limitation (EFL).

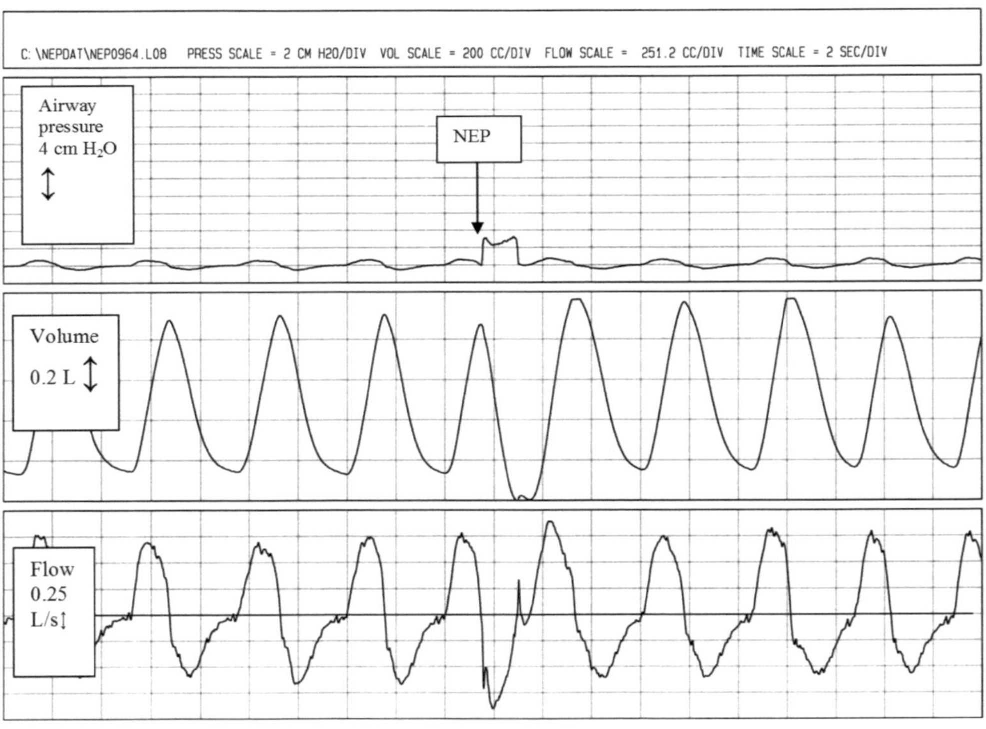

Figure 2. Tracings of airway pressure, volume and flow during quiet breathing. Application of negative expiratory pressure at the onset of expiration is indicated by NEP.

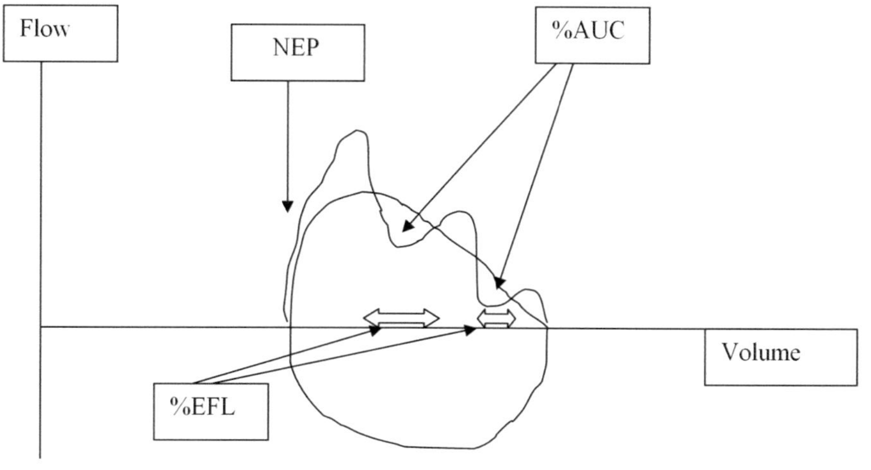

Figure 3. Schema of the control and NEP tidal flow-volume curves and how measurements of EFL% and AUC% were obtained.

As the driving pressure at the airway opening increases with application of NEP, expiratory flow should increase if the individual is not flow-limited (Figure 4).

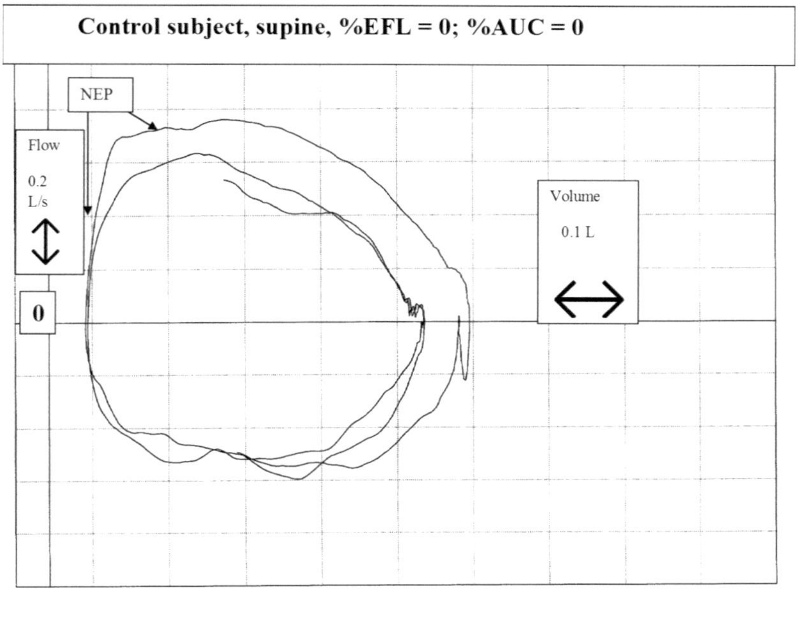

Figure 4. Tracings of the control and NEP tidal curves in a healthy subject. Note increase in expiratory flow with application of NEP.

By contrast, intrathoracic EFL is demonstrated by a sustained absence in increase in flow during application of NEP (as occurs in COPD) (Figure 5). That is, in these individuals the control and NEP-generated tidal expiratory are superimposed on each other.

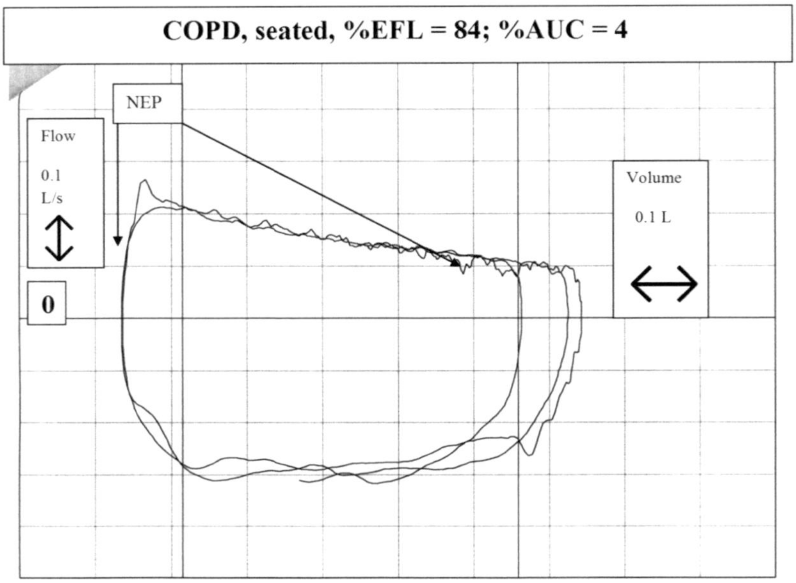

Figure 5. Tracings of control and NEP tidal curves in a patient with chronic obstructive pulmonary disease. Note absence of change in expiratory flow with application of NEP.

In obese individuals, some patients with restrictive respiratory disorders (Figure 6, individual with amyotrophic lateral sclerosis) and some subjects free of cardiorespiratory disease, application results in a reduction in the increase in flow or transient decrease below the control expiration. This finding is prevalent in patients with documented obstructive sleep apnea (Figure 7).

The NEP test is simple, noninvasive, practical and accurate. It has been validated by simultaneous determination of isovolume flow-pressure relationships (Valta et al., 1994).

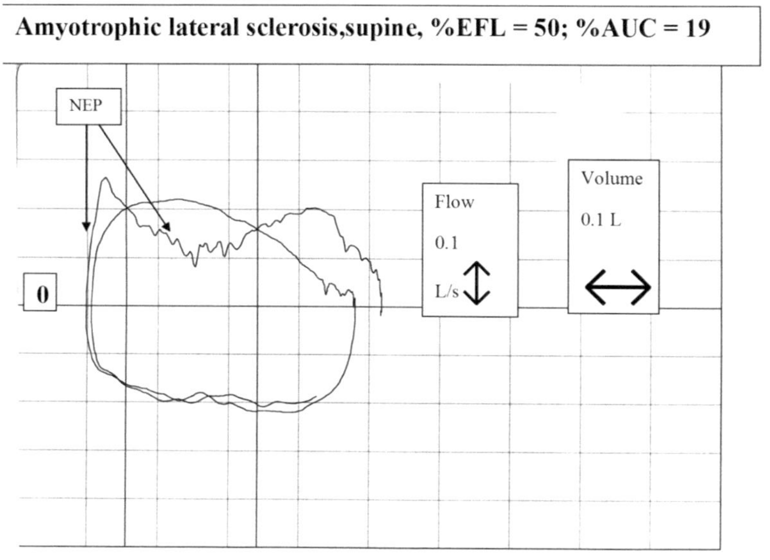

Figure 6. Tracings of control and NEP tidal flow-volume curves in a patient with a chest wall disorder, in this case amyotrophic lateral sclerosis with bulbar involvement (but without obstructive sleep apnea). Note the decrease in expiratory flow below the control tidal expiration with application of NEP.

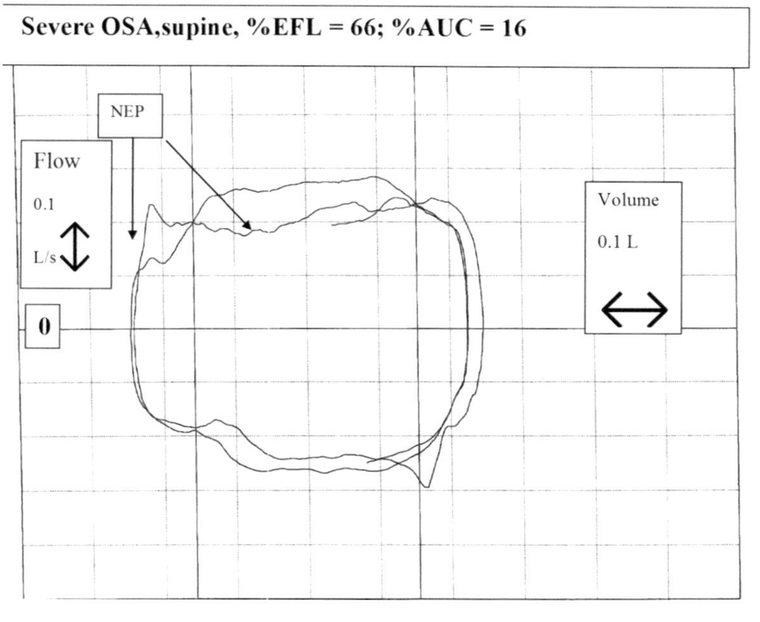

Figure 7. Tracings of control and NEP curves in a patient with severe obstructive sleep apnea. Note the sustained decrease of flow during application of NEP below the control expiratory tidal flow.

2.1. EFL in chronic obstructive pulmonary disease (COPD) and asthma

Fifty years ago, Hyatt (1961) suggested that patients with severe COPD may exhibit expiratory flow limitation (EFL) at rest. This phenomenon could be demonstrated by the finding that they breathed tidally along or above their maximal expiratory flow-volume curves. This pattern of tidal breathing leads to hyperinflation, increased work of breathing, impaired respiratory muscle function, hemodynamic compromise (Gottfried, 1991), and dyspnea (Eltayara et al., 1996; O'Donell et al., 1987). A high prevalence of tidal EFL is found in patients with COPD (Baydur et al., 2004; Gottfried et al., 1991; Hyatt et al., 1961) (Figure 5). As many as one-third of patients were flow-limited in seated and supine postures in the report of Baydur et al. (2004). A smaller percentage of patients with asthma in remission exhibit EFL, almost always in the supine posture (Baydur et al., 2004; Boczkowski et al., 1997).

The NEP technique can be used to advantage in young children unable to perform forced expiratory volume maneuvers (Braggion et al., 1998; Goetghebeur et al., 2002; Jiřičkova et al., 2009; Jones et al., 2000; Tauber, et al., 2003). Goetghebeur et al [10] described EFL in children aged older than 12 years with cystic fibrosis. These patients exhibited markedly decreased inspiratory capacity (IC) and forced expiratory volume at 1 sec (FEV_1). The NEP technique has also been used to evaluate EFL in infants (Braggion et al., 1998; Jiřičkova et al., 2009; Jones et al., 2000). Jiřičkova et al. (2009), applying the NEP technique in newborns and pre-school children, found nearly half of their patients to be intrathoracically flow-limited. The same number of children, however, exhibited transient upper airway collapse (UAC). The authors did not specify, if in some children, the UAC may have obscured any underlying intrathoracic EFL (see below).

An advantage of using the NEP technique in the evaluation of intrathoracic EFL is the avoidance of variability in the forced expiratory vital capacity maneuver related to the pattern of inspiratory maneuver preceding forceful expiration. Fast inspiration followed immediately by forced expiration results in greater forced vital capacities (FVC) and peak expiratory flows (PEF) by generating higher elastic recoil; in contrast, performing a breath-hold between inspiration and expiration diminishes elastic recoil and results in lower FVC and PEF. This finding, observed in both in healthy volunteers (D'Angelo et al., 1993; Tzelepis et al., 1997; Wanger et al., 1996) and patients (Braggion et al., 1996; D'Angelo et al., 1994; D'Angelo et al., 1996; Wanger et al., 1996), has been ascribed to the viscoelastic properties of the lung (D'Angelo et al., 1991) and to greater activation of expiratory muscles (Tzelepis et al., 1997) occurring with fast maneuvers. The NEP method also avoids underestimation of lung volumes during rapid expiratory maneuvers due to gas compression (Ingram & Schiller, 1966; Koulouris et al., 1995).The technique also avoids incorrect alignment of the tidal and maximal expiratory flow–volume curves. Such alignment is usually made considering the total lung capacity (TLC) as a fixed reference point, and this assumption may not always be valid (Kosmas et al., 2004; Koulouris, 1997; Murciano et al., 2000).

The NEP technique has also been used to detect EFL during exercise (Koulouris et al., 1997). In normal young subjects, there is no evidence of EFL during submaximal exercise. By contrast, most patients with COPD exhibit NEP-generated EFL during light exercise. These findings are in agreement with exercise studies employing conventional forced expiratory

http://dx.doi.org/10.5772/53270

flow-volume curves (Beck et al, 1991; Grimby & Stiksa, 1970; Hyatt, 1961; Kosmas et al., 2004; Koulouris, 1997; Murciano et al., 2000; Stubbing et al., 1980; Younes & Kivinen, 1984). Patients with EFL exhibit progressive lung inflation, increased sensation of dyspnea, and reduced maximal oxygen uptake during exercise.

Manual compression of the abdominal wall has also been used to detect EFL (Ninane et al., 2001). It has the advantage of generating an increase in abdominal pressure (of about 15 cm H_2O) that results in cranial displacement of the diaphragm into the thorax (provided it is relaxed) and a rise in pleural pressure (of about 6 cm H_2O) without the use of a special device. It also does not depend on previous volume and time history, and relies on a modest increase in alveolar pressure rather than a vacuum applied at the mouth, thus avoiding artifact caused by upper airway collapsibility. One study of this maneuver resulted in an increase in tidal expiratory flow in normal subjects, while it exhibited EFL in half of 12 patients with COPD in both supine and seated postures, and in 4 additional patients in supine position alone (Ninane et al., 2001).

Expiratory flow limitation is more prevalent in the elderly and is related to the severity of dyspnea (de Bisschop et al., 2005). In general, EFL does not closely correlate with FEV_1 or FEV_1/FVC (Eltayara et al., 1996). Older dyspneic individuals without cardiorespiratory disorders tend to be more flow limited than non-dyspneic persons (de Bisschop et al., 2005).

2.2. EFL in restrictive respiratory disorders

In individuals with restrictive disorders (particularly those with infiltrative disorders, such as idiopathic pulmonary fibrosis) maximal expiratory flows are well preserved despite a marked decrease in lung volume (Bergofsky, 1995). Consequently, breathing occurs at low lung volumes (near residual volume) where maximal expiratory flows are relatively small. Furthermore, some patients with interstitial lung diseases exhibit a decrease in dynamic compliance with breathing frequency (Bergofsky, 1995; Fulmer et al., 1977). In some of these patients, including non-smokers, flow rates are reduced with respect to transpulmonary pressure (Fulmer et al., 1977; Gaultier et al., 1980; Murphy et al., 38). Baydur et al. (1997, 2004) did not find any patients with restrictive disorders who exhibited intrathotracic EFL in either body position. The absence of EFL can be attributed to the increase in elastic recoil associated with these disorders. Others, however, have described the presence of EFL in patients with cardiac failure (Duguet et al., 2000), acute respiratory distress syndrome (Koutsoukou et al., 2000), and pleural effusions (Spyratos et al., 2007).

2.3. EFL in sleep apnea; differences in FL pattern from COPD and asthma as assessed by the NEP method

The NEP technique has also been used to assess upper airway collapsibility in patients with OSA, in which EFL has been described as a transient or sustained decrease in expiratory flow (frequently below the control tidal expiratory flow) during application of NEP (Baydur et al., 2004; Liistro et al., 1999; Van Meerhaeghe et al., 2004; Verin et al., 2002) (Figure 7).

Factors that contribute to OSA include increase in upper airway compliance (Isono et al., 1997), less negative critical (or closing) pressure of the passive upper airways as compared to snorers and normal subjects (related to structural soft tissue and bony changes) (Liistro et al., 1990), and smaller upper airway lumens during wakefulness and sleep, and greater pharyngeal airway length in OSA patients (Brown et al., 1985). Dyspnea in obese individuals is related to increased work of breathing related to decrease in FRC with resultant increase in intrathoracic EFL and intrinsic positive end-expiratory pressure, increased respiratory drive, and intermittent narrowing or collapse of the upper airway upon assuming the supine position (C.-K. Lin & C.-C. Lin, 2012).

Flow limitation can be assessed by computing the exhaled volume at specified time intervals during the application of NEP and expressed as percentage of the previous exhaled volume. Expiratory volumes at 0.2 and 0.5 sec after the application of NEP are significantly higher in awake healthy subjects than in awake patients with OSA (Insalaco et al., 2005; Romano et al., 2011). Expiratory volumes decline as disease severity increases., in these 2 studies, the exhaled volume at 0.2 sec exhibited a sensitivity, specificity, positive predictive value (PPV) and negative predictive value (NPV) to detect the presence of OSA of 81%, 93%, 98% and 53%, respectively (Insalaco et al., 2005; Romano et al., 2011). Sensitivity and negative predictive value both approached and reached 100% for moderate to severe [apnea-hypopnea index (AHI) 15-30], and severe (AHI >30) OSA, respectively. The authors concluded that FL measurements at 0.2 sec may be a useful screening test for suspected OSA (Insalaco et al., 2005; Romano et al., 2011).

Using a similar computational technique, Ferretti et al (2006) found that in awake OSA patients the exhaled volume during the first 0.5 sec after the onset of NEP averaged 20% and 31% less than snorers and control subjects, respectively, in supine posture (differences statistically significant). Under these conditions, an optimal cut-off value of 393 mL at NEP 0.5 sec exhibited a sensitivity, specificity, PPV and NPV of 76%, 74%, 84% and 64%, respectively. These differences were found to be less significant in the seated position. These authors concluded that while the NEP technique is potentially useful in evaluating upper airway collapsibility in OSA and its mechanisms while awake, it was not precise enough to differentiate simple snorers from those with OSA. Thus it cannot be recommended as a tool robust enough to screen obese patients or snorers for undergoing polysomnography (Ferretti et al., 2006).

2.3.1. Recent research by these authors

In patients with both COPD and OSA, EFL due to the intrathoracic component may be obscured by the presence of upper airway collapse or narrowing which frequently leads to a reduction in expiratory flow below that of the preceding control breath during application of NEP. Furthermore, distinguishing EFL in OSA from that of COPD can be problematic because patients may exhibit overlapping or combined EFL patterns combining features of both conditions. Baydur et al. (2012) compared the ability of the NEP technique to distinguish individuals with COPD from those with OSA and non-OSA obesity. EFL was quantitated using the following methods (Fig. 2):

http://dx.doi.org/10.5772/53270

1. EFL was expressed as percentage of the expired tidal volume over which the NEP-induced flow did not increase above the immediately preceding tidal expiratory flow (EFL%) (Baydur et al., 1997, 2004; Eltayara et al., 1996; Koulouris et al., 1995) for each subject in both postures as the median of 10 acceptable NEP breaths (Figure 3).

2. The magnitude of the decrease in expiratory flow during NEP below the preceding control expiratory curve was expressed as the percentage of the area under the control curve (AUC%, Figure 3), modified from the method of Tamisier et al. (2005). This value was expressed as the median of the same10 acceptable NEP breaths in each posture.

3. To further improve the discrimination between COPD and OSA, the ratio AUC% EFL% was computed as changes in EFL% and AUC% were not always of the same magnitude or direction. Thus, an increase AUC% EFL% would reflect a greater degree of upper airway EFL rather than intrathoracic EFL, while a decrease with preservation of EFL% would be more consistent with intrathoracic EFL. This quantity was expressed as an arbitrary unit, as the median of the same 10 acceptable NEP breaths in each posture.

This study was the first to quantitatively compare EFL in patients with COPD, non-OSA obesity and OSA in seated and supine postures. Its main findings were:

1. COPD patients exhibited the highest EFL% in seated posture, consistent with intrathoracic flow limitation. Percent EFL increased in all cohorts but COPD upon assuming the supine position.

2. While seated, when compared to other cohorts, OSA patients exhibited a greater tendency to upper airway collapsibility as evidenced by higher AUC% and AUC/% EFL% values, although median values exhibited variability of individual values that prevented differences between cohorts to be statistically significant. In supine posture, COPD patients exhibited the greatest AUC% but not AUC/% EFL.%

3. The AUC% method was able to only differentiate COPD patients from those with mild-moderate OSA in the seated position.

4. The AUC% method demonstrated higher AUC% in patients with OSA than in obese subjects, but was unable to clearly differentiate between the two groups because of overlapping values.

An increase in the AUC% and AUC/% EFL% reflects a greater degree of extrathoracic airflow limitation (as occurs in obese and OSA subjects) while an increase in EFL% in the absence of an increase in AUC% indicates the presence of intrathoracic flow limitation (as in COPD). Thus, subjects with greater increases in AUC/% EFL% than in EFL% upon assuming supine posture exhibit an increase in upper airway resistance rather than intrathoracic airflow limitation. At the same time, in patients with COPD, EFL% increases in supine position, a finding more likely to occur as FEV_1 decreases (Baydur et al., 1997, 2004; Eltayara et al., 1996; Koulouris et al., 1995).Variability in measurements using the NEP technique has been similarly reported by others (Hadcroft & Calverley, 2001; Walker et al., 2007) and is likely due to a number of factors, discussed below.

Percent AUC tended to be greater in OSA patients while seated indicating the presence of mechanisms maintaining upper airway patency while supine. By contrast, in COPD patients AUC% was greatest in supine posture, almost twice the value when seated. Thus, mechanisms preserving patency in supine COPD patients seem not to be as effective as in supine obese or OSA individuals. Reductions in lung volume (as occur in supine posture) result in decreases in caudal traction on the upper airway and concomitant increases in upper airway collapsibility (Owens et al., 2010; Squire et al., Thut et al., 1993; Van de Graaf, 1991). In addition, supine positioning promotes laryngeal edema and upper airway narrowing (Jafari & Mohsenin, 2011; Shepard et al., 1996). In COPD, mobilization of secretions when supine may have contributed to this finding. Yet, the finding of an overall increase in EFL% in supine position without concomitant increases in AUC% (or AUC/% EFL%) in most other cohorts indicated a greater degree of intrathoracic tidal EFL [as defined by Koulouris et al (1995)] than extrathoracic FL. This is likely related to decrease in lung volume when supine.)

The differing findings amongst cohorts can be explained thus: During early expiration, there is post-inspiratory inspiratory activity (PIIA) which may negate the effect of NEP. At the beginning of expiration, PIIA may oppose NEP (resistance posed by pliometric contraction [= lengthening] of the inspiratory muscles) (Shee et al., 1985). This implies that NEP should not be applied too early in expiration (when PIIA is high). In our subjects, NEP was applied immediately after the onset of expiratory flow so that PIIA is likely to have influenced variability of EFL within cohorts.

Our method for computing AUC% was similar to that of Tamisier et al. (2005) who devised a quantitative index corresponding to the ratio of the area under the expiratory flow-volume curves between NEP and control tidal volume. They did not, however, study subjects with mild OSA (BMI 5-15), and their control subjects were younger than ours. They also applied NEP near end-expiratory volume which stimulates activation of the genioglossus (Tantucci et al., 1998). This can change the area under the terminal portion of the NEP curve, affecting the quantitative index used to assess the upper airway collapsibility. Our results suggest that obese and OSA patients are more likely to experience upper airway narrowing while seated than COPD patients, indicating reduced PIIA and genioglossus activity in that posture.

There were some methodological limitations in this investigation. This study and those of others (Baydur et al., 2004, 2012; Insalaco et al., 2005; Liistro et al., 1999; Rouatbi et al., 2009; Van Meerhaeghe et al., 2004; Verin et al., 2002) assumed that upper airway collapsibility can be identified solely when expiratory flow during NEP decreases below the control curve. As such, detecting upper airway collapsibility only by computing the span of the preceding control tidal volume over which the NEP curve drops below the control breath may be misleading. It is possible that in this study some patients with upper airway narrowing may not have been identified if they exhibited only a reduction in the increase of expiratory flow (but still greater than the preceding control flow) during NEP.

Another limitation in this study was that sleep studies were not obtained in COPD patients and controls. Sleep-related disordered breathing (SDB) and nocturnal desaturations have been reported in COPD patients, giving rise to an "overlap syndrome" although not all SDB

http://dx.doi.org/10.5772/53270

could be classified as frank sleep apnea (Caterall et al., 1983; Aoki et al., 2005). Care was taken in this study, however, to exclude subjects with symptoms of sleep apnea. None of the obese COPD patients gave a history of symptoms of sleep apnea.

3. Conclusion

In conclusion, the EFL% and AUC% methods are useful in determining the magnitude of intrathoracic or extrathoracic FL in patients with COPD and OSA, but fail to distinguish cohorts on the basis of EFL quantification using the area under the curve method because of interindividual variabilities. In this respect, our findings were similar to those of Ferretti, et al. (2006). Pattern recognition of NEP tracings remains the best way to differentiate intrathoracic from extrathoracic EFL.

While the NEP method may be regarded as the new standard for the detection of tidal flow limitation (Koulouris, & Hardavella, 2011), further research should include its validation in conditions other than COPD that exhibit intrathoracic EFL. Comparison with other techniques such as the esophageal balloon, forced oscillation and abdominal compression (probably the easiest and least uncomfortable) methods should provide additional information in this regard. In the assessment of extrathoracic airway FL, the NEP technique offers a means to evaluate upper airway dynamics in patents with OSA, but is not able to differentiate snorers from those with OSA.

Acknowledgements

The authors thank Dr. Joseph Milic-Emili for valuable input to the manuscript; Mr. Louis Wilkinson for his valuable technical assistance; Dr. Danielle Kushner and Mr. Shadman Chowdhury for assistance in tabulating data. Dr. Cheryl Vigen and Dr. Zhanghua Chen provided critical statistical and data analysis. The authors also thank the technical staff of the Pulmonary Function Laboratory at Los Angeles County + University of Southern California Medical Center for performing the lung function and polysomnograhic testing, and all the patients and volunteers who participated in the study.

Abbreviation/Nomenclature list

AHI: Apnea-hypopnea index

AUC: Area under preceding control curve subtended by the NEP curve

BMI: Body mass index

EFL: Expiratory flow limitation

FEV_1: Forced expiratory volume in 1 second

FRC: Functional residual capacity

FVC: Forced vital capacity

AUC: Area under control tidal curve subtended by the immediately following NEP curve

NEP: Negative expiratory pressure

OSA: Obstructive sleep apnea

PEF: Peak expiratory flow

PIIA, post-inspiratory inspiratory activity

Vt: Tidal volume

Ti: Inspiratory time

Te: Expiratory time

TLC: Total lung capacity

Author details

Ahmet Baydur

Division of Pulmonary and Critical Care Medicine, Keck School of Medicine, University of Southern California, Los Angeles CA, USA

References

[1] Aoki, T., Ebihara, A., Salamaki, F., et al. (2005). Sleep disordered breathing in patients with chronic obstructive disease. *Journal of Chronic Obstructive Pulmonary Disease*, Vol. 2, pp. 243-252.

[2] Baydur, A. & Milic-Emili J. (1997). Expiratory flow limitation during spontaneous breathing: comparison of patients with restrictive and obstructive respiratory disorders. *Chest*, Vol. 112, pp. 1017-1023.

[3] Baydur, A., Vigen, C., Zhanghua, C. (2012). Expiratory flow limitation in obstructive sleep apnea and COPD: A quantitative method to detect pattern differences using the negative expiratory pressure technique. Accepted for publication, *The Open Respiratory Medical Journal*.

http://dx.doi.org/10.5772/53270

[4] Baydur, A., Wilkinson, L., Mehdian, R., Bains, B., Milic-Emili J. (2004). Extrathoracic expiratory flow limitation in obesity and obstructive and restrictive disorders. *Chest,* Vol. 125, pp. 98-105.

[5] Beck, K.C., Staets, B.A., Hyatt, R.E., Babb, T.G. (1991). Dynamics of breathing during exercise. In: *Exercise,* Whipp, B.J., Wasserman, K., (Eds.), pp. 67-97, Marcel Dekker, New York.

[6] Bergofsky, E.H. (1995). Thoracic deformities. In: *Lung Biology in Health and Disease. The Thorax, Part C: Disease,* Roussos C, (Ed.), pp. 1915-1949, Marcel Dekker, ISBN: 0-8247-9601-2, New York.

[7] Boczkowski, J., Murciano, D., Pichot, M.-H., Ferretti, A., Pariente, R., Milic-Emili, J. (1997). Expiratory flow-limitation in stable asthmatic patients during resting breathing. *American Journal of Respiratory and Critical Care Medicine,* Vol. 156, pp. 752-757, ISSN 1073-449X.

[8] Braggion, C., Polose, G., Fenzi, V., Carli, M.V., Pradal, U., Milic-Emili, J. (1998). Detection of tidal expiratory flow limitation in infants with cystic fibrosis. *Pediatriatric Pulmonology.* Vol. 25:213-215.

[9] Braggion, C., Pradal, G., Mastella, G., Coates, A., Milic-Emili, J. (1996). Effect of different inspiratory maneuvers on FEV_1 in patients with cystic fibrosis. *Chest,* Vol. 110, pp. 642-647.

[10] Brown, I.G., Bradley, T.D., Phillipson, E.A., Zamel, N., Hoffstein, V. (1985). Pharyngeal compliance in snoring subjects with and without obstructive sleep apnea. *American Journal of Respiratory and Critical Care Medicine,* Vol. 132, pp. 211-215, ISSN 1073-449X.

[11] Caterall, J.R., Douglas, N.J., Calverley, P.M., Shapiro, C.M., Brezinova, V., Brash, H.M. (1983). Transient hypoxemia during sleep in chronic obstructive pulmonary disease is not a sleep apnea syndrome. *American Journal of Respiratory and Critical Care Medicine,* Vol. 126, pp. 206-210, ISSN 00030805.

[12] D'Angelo, E., Milic-Emili, J., Marazzini, L. (1996). Effects of bronchodilator tone and gas density on time dependence of Forced expiratory vital capacity maneuver. *American Journal of Respiratory and Critical Care Medicine,* Vol. 154:1318-1322, ISSN 1073-449X.

[13] D'Angelo, E., Prandi, E., Milic-Emili, J. (1993). Dependence of maximal flow-volume curves on time course of preceding inspiration. *Journal of Applied Physiology,* Vol. 75, pp. 1155-1159.

[14] D'Angelo, E., Prandi, E., Marazzini, L., Milic-Emili, J. (1994). Dependence of maximal flow-volume curves on time course of preceding inspiration in patients with chronic obstructive pulmonary disease. *American Journal of Respiratory and Critical Care Medicine,* Vol. 150, pp. 1581-1586, ISSN 1073-449X.

[15] D'Angelo, E., Robatto, F.M., Calderini, E., Tavola, M., Bono, D., Torri, G., Milic-Emili, J. (1991). Pulmonary and chest wall mechanics in anesthetized paralyzed humans. *Journal of Applied Physiology,* Vol. 70, pp. 2602-2610.

[16] De Bisschop, C., Marty, M.L., Tessier, J.F., Barberger-Gateau, P., Dartigues, J.F., Guénard, H. (2005). Expiratory flow limitation and obstruction in the elderly. *European Respiratory Journal*. Vol. 26, pp. 594-601.

[17] Duguet, A., Tantucci, C., Lozinguez, O., Isnard, R., Thomas, D., Zelter, M., Derenne, J.-P., Milic-Emili, J., Expiratory flow limitation as a determinant of orthopnea in patients with acute left heart failure. *Journal of the American American College of Cardiology,* Vol. 35, pp. 690-700.

[18] Eltayara, L., Becklake, M.R., Volta, C.A., Milic-Emili, J. (1996). Relationship between chronic dyspnea and expiratory flow limitation in patients with chronic obstructive pulmonary disease. *American Journal of Respiratory and Critical Care Medicine,* Vol. 154, pp. 1726-1734.

[19] Ferretti, A., Giampiccolo, P., Redolfi, S., Mondini, S., Cirignotta, F., Cavalli, A., Tantucci, C. (2006). Upper airway dynamics during negative expiratory pressure in apneic and non-apneic awake snorers. *Respiratory Research,* Vol. 7, pp. 54-64. doi: 10.1186/1465-9921-7-54.

[20] Fulmer, J.D., Roberts, W.C., von Gal, E.R., Crystal, R.G. (1977). Small airways in idiopathic pulmonary fibrosis. *Journal of Clinical Investigation,* Vol. 60, pp. 595-610. PMCID: PMC372404.

[21] Gaultier, G., Chaussain, M., Boule, M., et al. (1980). Lung function in interstitial lung diseases in children. *Bulletin Europeén Physiopathologie Respiratoire,* Vol. 16, pp. 57-66.

[22] Goetghebeur, D., Sarni, D., Grossi, Y., Leroyer, C., Ghezzo, H., J., M. Bellet, M. (2002). Tidal expiratory flow limitation and chronic dyspnea in patients with cystic fibrosis. *European Respiratory Journal,* Vol. 19, pp. 492-498.

[23] Gottfried, S.B. (1991). The role of PEEP in the mechanically ventilated COPD patient. In: *Ventilatory Failure,* Marini, J.J., Roussos, C. (Eds.), pp. 392–418, Springer-Verlag, Berlin.

[24] Grimby, G. & Stiksa, J. (1970). Flow-volume curves and breathing patterns during exercise in patients with obstructive lung disease. *Scandinavian Journal of Clinical and Laboratory Investigation,* Vol. 25, pp. 303-313.

[25] Hadcroft, J. & Calverley, P.M.A. (2001). Alternative methods for assessing bronchodilator reversibility in chronic obstructive pulmonary disease. *Thorax,* Vol. 56, pp. 713-720.

[26] Hyatt, R.E. (1961). The interrelationship of pressure, flow and volume during various respiratory maneuvers in normal and emphysematous patients. *American Review of Respiratory Disease,* Vol. 83, pp. 676-683.

[27] Ingram, R.H., Schiller, P.D. (1966). Effect of gas compression on the flow-volume curve of the forced vital capacity. *American Review of Respiratory Disease,* Vol. 94, pp. 56-63.

[28] Insalaco, G., Romano, S., Marrone, O., Salvaggio, A., Bonsignore, G. (2005). A new method of negative expiratory pressure test analysis detecting upper airway flow limitation to reveal obstructive sleep apnea. *Chest,* Vol. 128: 2159-2165.

[29] Isono, S, Remmers, J.E., Tanaka, A., Sho, Y., Sato, J., Nishino, T. (1997). Anatomy of pharynx in patients with obstructive sleep apnea and in normal subjects. *Journal of Applied Physiology,* Vol. 82, pp. 1319-1326.

[30] Jafari, B., Mohsenin, V. (2011). Overnight rostral fluid shift in obstructive apnea. *Chest,* Vol. 140, pp. 991-997.

[31] Jiřičkova, A., Šulc, J., Pohunek, P., Kittnar, O., Dohnalová, A., Kofránek, J. (2009). Prevalence of tidal expiratory flow limitation in preschool children with and without respiratory symptoms: Application of the negative expiratory pressure (NEP) method. *Physiological Research,* Vol. 58, pp. 373-382.

[32] Jones, M.H., Davis, S.D., Kisling, J.A., Howard, J.M., Castile, R., Tepper, R.S. (2000). Flow limitation in infants assessed by negative expiratory pressure. *American Journal of Respiratory and Critical Care Medicine,*Vol. 161, pp. 713-717.

[33] Kosmas, E.N., Milic-Emili, J., Polychronaki, A., Dimitroulis, I., Retsou, S., Gaga, M. , Koutsoukou, A., Roussos, Ch., N.G. Koulouris, N.G. (2004). Exercise-induced flow limitation, dynamic hyperinflation and exercise capacity in patients with bronchial asthma. *European Respiratory Journal,* Vol. 24, pp. 378-384.

[34] Koulouris, N.G., Dimopoulou, I., Valta, P., Finkelstein, R., Cosio, M.G., Milic-Emili, J. (1997). Detection of expiratory flow limitation during exercise in COPD patients. *Journal of Applied Physiology,* Vol. 82, pp. 723-731.

[35] Koulouris, N.G. & Hardavella, G. (2011). Physiological techniques for detecting expiratory flow limitation during tidal breathing. *European Respiratory Journal*, Vol. 20, pp. 147–155. ISSN 0905-9180.

[36] Koulouris, N.G., Valta, P., Lavoie, A., Corbeil, C., Chassé, M., Braidy, J, Milic-Emili, J. (1995). A simple method to detect expiratory flow limitation during spontaneous breathing. *European Respiratory Journal,* Vol. 8, pp. 306-313.

[37] Koutsoukou, A., Armaganidis, A., Stavrakaki-Kallergi, C., Vassilakopoulos, T., Lymberis, A., Roussos, C., Milic-Emili, J. (2000). Expiratory flow limitation and intrinsic positive end-expiratory pressure at zero positive end-expiratory pressure in patients with adult respiratory distress syndrome. *American Journal of Respiratory and Critical Care Medicine,* Vol. 161, pp. 1590-1596.

[38] Liistro, G., Stanescu, D., Dooms, G., Veriter, C., Aubert-Tulkens, G., Rodenstein, D. (1990). Hypopharyngeal and neck cross-sectional changes monitored by inductive plethysmography. *Journal of Applied Physiology,* Vol. 68, pp. 2649-2655.

[39] Liistro, G., Veriter, C., Dury, M., Aubert, G., Stanescu, D. (1999). Expiratory flow-limitation in awake sleep- disordered breathing subjects. *European Respiratory Journal,* Vol. 14, pp. 185-190.

[40] Lin C-K, Lin C-C. (2012). Work of breathing and respiratory drive in obesity. *Respirology* Vol. 17, pp. 402-411.

[41] Murciano, D., Ferretti, A., Boczkowski, J., Sleiman, C., Fournier, M., Milic-Emili, J. (2000). Flow limitation and dynamic hyperinflation during exercise in COPD patients after single lung transplantation. *Chest,* Vol. 118, pp. 1248-1254, ISSN: 0012-3692.

[42] Murphy, D.M.F., Hall, D.R., Petersen, M.R., Lapp, N.L. (1981). The effect of diffuse pulmonary fibrosis on lung mechanics. *Bulletin Europeen Physiopathologie Respiratoire,* Vol. 17, pp. 27-41.

[43] Ninane, V., Leduc, D., Abdel Kafi, S., Nasser, M., Houa, M., Sergysels, R. (2001). Detection of expiratory flow limitation by manual compression of the abdominal wall. *American Journal of Respiratory and Critical Care Medicine,* Vol. 163, pp. 1326-1330.

[44] O'Donell, D.E., Sanii, R., Anthonisen, N.R., Younes, M. (1987). Effect of dynamic airway compression on breathing pattern and respiratory sensation in severe chronic obstructive pulmonary disease. *American Journal of Respiratory and Critical Care Medicine,* Vol. 135, pp. 912-918.

[45] Owens, R.L., Malhotra, A., Eckert, D.J., White, D.P., Jordan, A.S. (2010). The influence of end-expiratory lung volume on measurements of pharyngeal collapsibility. *Journal of Applied Physiology,* Vol. 108, pp. 445-451.

[46] Romano, A., Salvaggio, A., Lo Bue, A., Marrone, O., Insalaco, G. (2011). A negative expiratory pressure test during wakefulness for evaluating the risk of obstructive sleep apnea in patients referred for sleep studies. *Clinics (Sao Paulo),* Vol. 66, pp. 1887-1894 , 22086518.

[47] Rouatbi, S., Tabka, Z., Dogui, M., Abdelghani, A., Guénard, H. (2009). Negative expiratory pressure (NEP) parameters can predict obstructive sleep apnea syndrome in snoring patients. *Lung,* Vol. 187, pp. 23-28.

[48] Shee, C.D., Ploy-song-sang, Y., Milic-Emili, J. (1985). Decay of inspiratory muscle pressure during expiration in conscious humans. *Journal of Applied Physiology,* Vol. 58, pp. 1859-1865.

[49] Shepard, J.W. Jr., Pevernagie, D.A., Stanson, A.W., Daniels, B.K., Sheedy, P.F. (1996). Effects of changes in central venous pressure on upper airway size in patients with obstructive sleep apnea. *American Journal of Respiratory and Critical Care Medicine,* Vol. 153, pp. 250-254.

[50] Spyratos, D., Sichletidis, L., Manika, K., Kontakiotis, T., Chloros, D., Patakas, D. (2007). Expiratory flow limitation in patients with pleural effusion. *Respiration,* Vol. 74, pp. 572-578.

[51] Squire, S.B., Patil, S.P., Schneider, H., Kirkness, J.P., Smith, P.L. (2010). Effect of end-expiratory lung volume on upper airway collapsibility in sleeping men and women. *Journal of Applied Physiology,* Vol. 109, pp. 977-985.

[52] Stubbing, D.G., Pengelly,L.D., Morse, J.L.C., Milic-Emili, J. (1980). Pulmonary mechanics during exercise in subjects with chronic airflow obstruction. *Journal of Applied Physiology,* Vol. 49, pp. 511–515.

[53] Tamisier, R., Wuyam, B., Nicolle, I., Pepin, J.L., Orliaguet, O., Perrin, C.P., Levy, P. (2005). Awake flow limitation with negative expiratory pressure in sleep disordered breathing. *Sleep Medicine,* Vol. 6, pp. 205-213.

[54] Tantucci, C., Mehiri, S., Duguet, A., Similowski, T., Arnulf, I., Zelter, M., Derenne, J.-P., Milic-Emili, J. (1998). Application of negative expiratory pressure during expiration and activity of genioglossus in humans. *Journal of Applied Physiology,* Vol. 84, pp. 1076-1082.

[55] Tauber, E., Fazekas, T., Eichler, I., Eichstill, C., Partner, C., Koller, D.Y., Fischer, T. (2003). Negative expiratory pressure: A new tool for evaluating lung function in children? *Pediatric Pulmonology,* Vol. 35, pp. 162-168.

[56] Thut, D.C., Schwartz, A.R., Roach, D., Wise, R.A., Permutt, S., Smith, P.L. (1993). Tracheal and neck position influence upper airway flow dynamics by altering airway length. *Journal of Applied Physiology,* Vol. 75, pp. 2084-2090.

[57] Tzelepis, G.E., Zakynthinos, S., Vassilakopoulos, T., Geroulanos, S., Roussos, C. (1997). Inspiratory maneuver effects on peak expiratory flow: Role of lung elastic recoil and expiratory pressure. *American Journal of Respiratory and Critical Care Medicine,* Vol. 156, pp. 1399-1404.

[58] Valta, P., Corbeil, C., Lavoie, A., Campodonico, R., Koulouris, N., Chassé, M., Braidy, J., Milic-Emili, J. (1994). Detection of expiratory flow limitation during mechanical ventilation. *American Journal of Respiratory and Critical Care Medicine,* Vol. 150, pp. 1311-1317.

[59] Van de Graaff, W.B. (1991). Thoracic traction on the trachea: mechanisms and magnitude. *Journal of Applied Physiology,* Vol. 70, pp. 1328-1336.

[60] Van Meerhaeghe, A., Delpire, P., Stenuit, P., Kerkhofs, M. (2004). Operating characteristics of the negative expiratory pressure technique in predicting obstructive sleep apnoea syndrome in snoring patients. *Thorax* Vol. 59, pp. 883-888.

[61] Verin, E., Tardif, C., Portier, F., Similowski, T., Pasquis, P., Muir, J.F. (2002). Evidence for expiratory flow limitation of extrathoracic origin in patients with obstructive sleep apnoea. *Thorax,* Vol. 57, pp. 423-428.

[62] Walker, R., Paratz, J., Holland, A.E. (2007). Reproducibility of the negative expiratory pressure technique in COPD. *Chest,* Vol. 132, pp. 471-476.

[63] Wanger., J.S., Ikle, D.N., Cherniack, R.M. (1996). The effect of inspiratory maneuvers on expiratory flow rates in health and asthma: influence of lung elastic recoil. *American Journal of Respiratory and Critical Care Medicine,* Vol. 153, pp. 1302-1308.

[64] Younes, M. & Kivinen, G. (1984). Respiratory mechanics and breathing pattern during and following maximal exercise. *Journal of Applied Physiology,* Vol. 57: 1773–1782.

Section 3

Parasitic Tropical Lung Diseases

Chapter 7

Tropical Lung Diseases

Ntumba Jean-Marie Kayembe

Additional information is available at the end of the chapter

http://dx.doi.org/10.5772/52371

1. Introduction

Infectious disease results from the disruption of the balance between the host and the pathogen. Pathogen influencing factors include virulence, immunoevasion capacities, and drug resistance ability. According to the host, disease outcome relay on many factors such as: immunocompetence, comorbidities, terrain (ageing, malnutrition).

The lung epithelium is a large surface exposed to outside aggression. The environment plays a key role in the onset and development of illness by many factors such as: climate, social and cultural habits, vegetations, degree of industrial, or domestic pollutions...

Despite this exaggerated exposition, the lung is nevertheless protected through non specific and/ or specific defense mechanisms (Agostini CV, Chilosi M, Zambello R et *al*, 1993).

1.1. Non specific defense mechanisms

According to its size, a foreign substance can reach the upper or lower respiratory tract, and be cleaned via the mucociliary escalator, during coughing or sneezing. Epithelial cells also secrete many agents such as lysozyme, toxic oxygen radicals, with antimicrobial properties. The renewal of the epithelium, as for the skin, is an additional protecting property.

Innate immune recognition is a second protective mechanism implicating immune cells and secreted mediators. Its under the control of cells carrying receptors for recognition of foreign antigens (PRRs: pathogen recognition receptors) such as macrophages, dendritic cells, neutrophils, mastocytes, epithelial cells, NK cells, and fibroblasts which can link microbial structures (PAMPS: pathogen associated molecular patterns) for further destruction (Ahnen DJ, 1985).

1.2. Specific defense mechanisms

Adaptive immunity relays on the interaction between antigen-presenting cells (macrophages, dendritic cells, neutrophils) with specific T-lymphocytes in the context of cell mediated immunity, as well as, on the antibodies production by activated B-lymphocytes (humoral immunity) (Kohlmeter JE, Woodland DL, 2006).

2. Tropical parasitic lung diseases

2.1. Overview

Protozoa and helminthes can affect the lung as a primary site, or a complication. Some parasites have a migration cycle through the lung (larva migrans), inducing blood and tissue eosinophilia. Tissue and peripheral blood eosinophilia are elicited by chimiotactic activity of released inflammatory mediators, such as cytokines (IL-3, IL-5), which play a key role in activation and differentiation of eosinophils. Eosinophils secrete various substances, some with antiparasitis properties, others favoring tissue damage in targeted organs. Elevated IgE level observed in these conditions relay on the Th2-lymphocytes, stimulating antibodies production by B-lymphocytes (Om P Sharma, 1991; VijayanVK, 2008).

Clinical manifestations of the lung involvement could be acute: asthma –like syndrome, or Loeffler's syndrome, with dyspnea, wheezing, cough (Ford RM, 1996); or chronic such as hemoptysis or right heart failure signs. Acute manifestations depend on immunological reaction (hypersensitivity), and chronic feature relay on the mechanical action of pathogen on the vessels and tissues. (vg: schistosoma eggs in the pulmonary artery and pulmonary hypertension). (Santiago M et *al.*, 2005).

Löeffler's syndrome represent transient clinical, immunological and radiological manifestations due to parasites whose life cycle elicit a transit through the lung or not, and to drug reactions

Hypereosinophilia observed in this syndrome is antigen –induced, and circulating IL-5, is the key mechanism for the recruitment and differentiation of the eosinophils.

2.2. Helminthic parasites

The three classes of helminths (Cestoidea, Trematoda, and Nematoda) can affect the lung.

2.2.1. Nematodes and the lung

This group include: ascariasis, strongyloidiasis,ancylostomiasis, tropical pulmonary eosinophilia, pulmonary dirofilariasis, and pulmonary trichinellosis.

2.2.1.1. Pulmonary ascariasis

Ascariasis is a round worm infection caused by Ascaris lumbricoides. This nematode disease affects ± 25% of the world population whose 95% are in Africa (Crompton, 1999).

http://dx.doi.org/10.5772/52371

Mode of contamination

The starting point is the survival of eggs able to contaminate ingesta by the new host. Poor sanitation, fecal contamination of food or water, are the main risk factors of dissemination. Embryonated eggs (2-4 weeks), when ingested are dissolved in the stomach juice and then release rabdoid larvae in the duodenum, before migration through the intestine. Larvae then enter the portal system via capillaries and lymphatics, after penetrating the wall of the intestine. The involvement of the hepatic circulation allow the right heart and lung invasion. The eggs reach the alveolar space after crossing the capillary walls and can be swallowed and then reach again the small intestine to mute in adult forms. This pilgrimage can take 14 days after ingestion (Sarinas PS, Chitkara RK, 1997).

Pathophysiology

Adult worms or migrating larvae exert a mechanical pressure on lung structures inducing inflammatory responses, leading to granuloma formation with eosinophils, neutrophils and macrophages. Activated cells release cytokines such as IL-3 and IL-5 involved in the recruitment and differenciation of eosinophils, explaining the blood and tissue eosinophilia reported. TH2 Lymphocytes are responsible for the high IgE (Yazicioglia, 1996) and IgG4 levels (Santra A, 2001) described.

Hypersensitivity reaction inducing peribronchial inflammation, mucus production, and sometimes bronchospasm is responsible for the clinical manifestations.

Diagnosis

Abdominal manifestations are currently reported: gastric pain, vomiting, diarrhea, abdominal discomfort. In some complicated cases pancreatitis or obstruction of biliary duct or small intestine can occur, caused by adult worms.

Respiratory symptoms due to larval migration in the lungs, consist in mild cough or Loeffler's syndrome (Ford RM, 1996). This syndrome associates respiratory symptoms (dry cough, wheezing, dyspnoea) with blood and lung eosinophilia, and chest radiograph with fleeting infiltrates. General symptoms such as fever, loss of appetite, myalgia can be observed.

Pneumonia is a more rare condition with ascariasis infection

Laboratory findings

Stool examination may show eggs or adult worms.

Larvae may be found in respiratory secretions

Serological approach (specific IgG4 antibodies) could be helpful (Santra A *et al.*, 2001; Bhattacharya T, 2001).

Blood hypereosinophilia and high IgE level are common.

Chest radiograph may show migrating inhomogenous alveolar infiltrates.

Treatment

The treatment aims to eradicate intestinal colonization responsible for recurrent respiratory episodes.

Mebendazole (100 mg twice a day for three days, or 500mg one day) and Albendazole (400mg, single dose) are the drugs of choice. Pyrantel Pamoate, Levamisole, and Piperazine are alternative choices. Ivermectine, an antifilarial drug has shown efficacy in the treatment of ascariasis.

2.2.1.2. Toxocariasis

a roundworm of dog and cat can infect human, who is an intermediate host, and determine a Loeffler's like syndrome caused by larva migrans as with Ascaris.

Severe respiratory syndromes (ARDS) have rarely been observed (Bartelink AK et *al.*, 1983), while asthma-like symptoms are currently reported among pulmonary manifestations.

Defects in neutrophil function have been reported in children with visceral larva migrans. This defect should be explained by the neutrophilic adherence to larvae illustrated elsewhere in animal models (Martin Huwer, 1989).

Exacerbations of inflammatory reactions during antihelminthic treatment emphasize the need of combination with corticosteroids.

2.2.1.3. Pulmonary strongyloidiasis

The causative agent is Strongyloides stercoralis, endemic in the tropics and subtropics. Eggs containing larvae ready to hatch, are the contaminating form after penetrating the skin; they then disseminate in all tissues via venous or lymphatic route in immunodeficient host (Cook, 1987; Longworth and Weller, 1986).

Autoinfestation is a common feature of this parasite, meaning the penetration of filariform larvae in the perianal skin of the infected subject without leaving the host. This phenomenon can determine the persistence of infection even many years after (Scowden EB, 1978).

Lung invasion result from larvae carried by the blood stream to the right heart and then to the lung. Larvae can pierce the pulmonary capillaries and reach the alveoli through the alveolo-capillary membrane, inducing non cardiogenic edema and hemoptyses. After their migration through the bronchi and superior respiratory tree, some larvae can be swallowed in the intestine. Hyperinfection syndrome is related to severity of symptoms in the lung and the intestine, which are common sites of the parasitic life cycle, while disseminated disease represent the invasion of other organs not generally involved in the growth of the parasite (Longoworth DL, and Weller PF, 1986).

Pathophysiology

The skin penetration by the larva determines an hypersensitivity reaction as the result of a strong cell mediated immunity reaction in immunocompetent host preventing the tissue invasion (Neva FA, 1986). Marked autoinfection and subsequent hyperinfection are the main determinants of tissue dissemination in immunosuppressed subjects such as AIDS patients

http://dx.doi.org/10.5772/52371

(Lessman KD, 1993), individuals on long term corticosteroid therapy, or with malnutrition, lymphomas etc..(Casati A, 1996; Genta RM, 1989).

Mechanical action by the adult worms and host reaction are responsible for digestive manifestations.

Secondary gram negative bacterial infection by gram- pathogen is frequent, bacteria being carried by larvae during the crossing of the intestinal wall. The migration through the lung can determine bronchopneumonia,alveolar hemorrhages, and pulmonary abscess and haemoptyses.

Diagnosis

Lung strongyloidiasis is commonly asymptomatic in immunocompetant individuals, or present with mild symptoms.

Gastrointestinal manifestations, cough, dyspnoea, wheezing and haemoptysis are frequent during lung involvement. Hyperinfection and disseminated disease are commonly fatal, which elderly individuals and those on long term corticosteroid therapy, or having hematologic malignancies being at higher risk for the latter.

Eosinophilic pleural effusion have been reported among pulmonary manifestations of strongyloidiasis; and rare cases of acute respiratory failure due to respiratory muscle paralysis have been observed (da Silva OA, 1981).

The hyperinfection syndrome with Strongyloides stercoralis can worsen asthma or COPD exacerbations in some patients (Sen P, 1995; Ossorio MA, 1990).

Peripheral blood eosinophilia, anemia, and hypoalbuminemaia are current laboratory findings.

Larva may be observed in repeted stool specimen examination due to the low parasitic load in immunocompetent individuals.

Pulmonary secretions, duodenal juice, may be contributive for parasite identification.

Serology is also interesting for detection of specific antibodies.

Treatment

Thiabendazole (25 mg/kg, twice a day for two days), Albendazole (400 mg, twice a day/5 days), Ivermectine (200 microgr/kg for one or two days) are recommended.

2.2.1.4. Pulmonary ancylostomiasis

Ancylostoma duodenale and *Necator americanus* are the two helminths in this group.

Eggs eliminated with the feces continue the maturation in the soil, where larvae will penetrate the intact skin to infect the man, which is the only definitive host. The oral route of infection is possible for *Ancylostoma duodenale*. Migrant larvae reach the lung structures has illustrate for other helminths, inducing a Loeffler's syndrome. The larvae of *Ancylostoma du-*

odenale can reach the mammary glands and be transmitted to the child by maternal breast-feeding (Yu Sen-Hai, 1995).

Pathophysiology

The lung migration can elicit blood eosinophilia as for other larva migrans. Larvae release low molecular weight proteins with anticoagulant properties (Cappello M, 1993), favoring blood loss during the intestinal capillaries destruction. Anemia with iron deficiency is often associated with this infection.

Local prurit and erythema follow skin penetration. Clinical, immunological and radiological manifestations of Loeffler's syndrome can be observed during larval migration through the lung.

Diagnosis

Gastrointestinal symptoms associated with respiratory asthma-like symptoms in an exposed individual are suggestive of parasitic lung infections

Laboratory findings

Stool examination may demonstrate the presence of eggs, blood samples may identify eosinophilia and iron deficient anemia.

Treatment

Mebendazole and Albendazole have equivalent efficacy.

Ivermectine has been reported as an alternative.

2.2.1.5. Tropical Pulmonary Eosinophilia (TPE)

This syndrome is an immunological response of the host to filarial parasites invasion, mainly Wuchereria bancrofti and Brugia malayi, affecting only 1% of patients with filariasis (Johnson S, 1994).

The filarial etiology has been suggested by the prevalent occurrence of the syndrome in the world regions with reported high filarialsis prevalence (South-East Asia), as well as the recovery after antifilarial drug administration.

Pathophysiology

The hypersensitivity reaction to filarial antigens induce a strong eosinophilic inflammatory response in the lungs. The microfilariae in lymphatics invade the pulmonary circulation and parenchyma with further granulomatous and fibrosing pattern. The concentration of eosinophils in the lung has been shown to be more significant than in the peripheral blood suggesting the compartimentalisation, and a prominent role of these cells in the pulmonary involvement and clinical manifestations (Pinkstori P, 1987).

Diagnosis

Epidemiological data state a male predominance in TPE (sex ratio M/F; 4:1), a disease of children and young adult (15-40 yrs).

http://dx.doi.org/10.5772/52371

Respiratory manifestations are frequently associated with systemic symptoms such as: fever, weight loss, and fatigue.

The diagnosis should be evoked after exclusion of other causes of pulmonary eosinophilia as other helmintic diseases, or drug use.

Laboratory findings

Leucocytosis is common in TPE, with marked peripheral blood eosinophilia; and elevated erythrocyte sedimentation rate is often reported.

Serological examinations may reveal high level of specific IgG or IgE antibodies to microfilariae.

Stool examination is very important to determine co-infection with other helminths.

The chest radiograph may show miliairy nodules mimicking miliairy tuberculosis.

Histopathological analysis of lung biopsies may illustrate microfilariae

Treatment

Diethylcarbamazine (6 mg/kg/day for 3 weeks), a current treatment of filariasis, has been successfully indicated In patients with TPE.

Steroids have shown additional improvement of symptoms in TPE patients.

2.2.1.6. Pulmonary dirofilariasis

This is a zoonosis caused by Dirofilaria immitis and repens. The nematode is a vascular parasite, with the human as accidental host. The parasite is transmitted by mosquito. The vascular location induce embolism of pulmonary artery, with subsequent pathophysiological manifestations such as: hemoptyses, chest pain, dyspnoea ...

The disease is mainly asymptomatic

Thoracic imaging (TTDM) shows well delimited nodule neigbouring an arterial branch.

Histopathological analysis of pulmonary biopsies is strongly contributive for the diagnosis of this disease lacking specific treatment.

2.2.1.7. Pulmonary Trichinellosis

The food-borne disease is caused by *Trichinella spiralis* in the man.

The larvae grow in striated muscles after invading the bloodstream. Man is infected after ingesting partially or cooked or raw meat, and the larvae develop in the gut into adult worms.

Pulmonary symptoms include: dyspnoea due partially to the involvement of diaphragm, and cough.

Peripheral blood eosinophilia and elevated IgE level are depending on Th-2 cytokines released by TCD4 cells recruited by parasitic antigens. Elevated LDH enzyme suggest muscle involvement.

Larvae may be also identified in striated muscle biopsies.

Treatment

Mebendazole (for almost 2 weeks), associated to analgesics and corticosteroids is recommended.

2.2.1.8. CESTODES and the lung

Lung disease due to cestodes are caused by *Echinococcus granulosis* and *Echinococcus multilocularis* in the man. The lung and the liver are the main sites of cysts formation. Dogs are definitive hosts and eggs excreted in their faeces contaminate human when ingested with food or water.

Pulmonary symptoms are non specific and resemble asthma manifestations. Mechanical compression by hydatid cysts may influence clinical features. Rupture of Cysts in the bronchi could explain haemoptysis or excretion of cyst fluid, and may lead to anaphylaxis. Pneumothorax, pleural effusion, and emphysema are possible lung presentation.

Blood laboratory findings extend from eosinophilia to IgE production.

Serodiagnosis is helpful by detection of specific antibodies.

Chest radiograph manifestations may consist in multiple nodules mimicking lung tumors.

Treatment

Surgical resection of the lesion is the most relevant approach. Mebendazole, Albendazole and praziquantel are indicated, mainly in recurrent disease.

2.2.1.9. Trematodes and the lung

This group include pulmonary scistosomiasis and paragonimiasis.

Pulmonary Shistosomiasis

Schistosoma haematobium, mansoni, and *japonicum* are the major pathogenic species for human. *Shistosoma intercalatum* and *Shistosoma mekongi* are rarely encountered. Eggs excreted in urine or faeces of the infected patient contaminate water and infect the snail, intermediate host. The eggs then evolve in cercariae wich can penetrate the skin or be ingested by man. The adult worm stay in the bladder (*haematobium*), or in the gut (*S. mansoni, S. japonicum*).

Pathophysiology

Local inflammation occurs at the penetration site, while the onset of pulmonary manifestations may be acute or chronic.

Pulmonary inflammatory reaction may induce a cytotoxic reaction to migrating agents, and facilitate the secretions of chimiotactic mediators for eosinophils, involved in the *schistosoma* immunity (Schwartz E et *al*, 2000).

Acute manifestations result from immunologic hypersensitivity reactions, and consist of systemic complaints such as fever, myalgia, chills, diarrhea, abdominal pain, urticaria,

http://dx.doi.org/10.5772/52371

named Katayama syndrome. Pulmonary acute manifestations mimic Loffler's syndrome or Asthma-like syndrome (Walt F., 1954).

Chronic manifestations result from mechanical action of eggs or adult worm on the tissues. Pulmonary hypertension, haemoptysis, cor pulmonale could be observed. Pulmonary embolism is the consequence of small blood vessels obstruction by foreign bodies surrounded by various cells (eosinophils, neutrophils, lymphocytes, giant multinucleated cells (Wyler and Postlehwaite WE, 1983); Granuloma formation is the end-stage of the maintained inflammatory response to schistosomal antigens.

Optic microscopical identification of eggs in urine or stools is mandatory for the diagnosis. Rectal or bladder's mucosal biopsies could help demonstrating eggs of Schistosoma.

Extrapulmonary manifestations include hepatosplenomegaly due to portal hypertension. Schistosomiasis is an infectious cause of liver cirrhosis.

Peripheral blood eosinophilia and high IgE level are frequent.

Treatment

Cortcosteroides are indicate during acute phase and praziquantel (10-15 mg/kg, each 12 hours, one day). Artemether has shown effectiveness on juvenile forms of schistosomes.

Pulmonary Paragonimiasis

The food-borne zoonosis is more frequent in Asia, affecting± 20 million people (Schwartz E, 2002); Subacute or chronic lung manifestations are described. The agent Paragonimus westermani lives in the lung, and eggs are eliminated in the sputum or faeces. Miracidiae develop into cercariae in the snail before infecting the second intermediate host, the crabs. The man get infection after eating partially cooked or raw crabs.

Clinical manifestations are not specific, and chest radiograph may demonstrate cavitations as in tuberculosis. Pleural effusion or pneumothorax are frequently seen in paragonimiasis.

Treatment

Praziquantel is the first choice for treatment of this helminthic disease.

2.3. Protozoal lung diseases

2.3.1. Pulmonary amoebiasis

Entamoeba histolytica is the pathogenic form of infectious agent for the man.

Lung involvement is mainly linked to extension of amoebic liver abscess; hematogenous spread and aspiration have rarely been reported (Shamsuzzaman SM et *al*, 2002).

During intestinal transit and mutations, Trophozoites released after the cysts digestion by digestive secretions, may reach the muscularis mucosa and erode the lymphatics or the walls of mesenteric venules to invade the portal system of the liver. The parasitic embols then obstruct the bloodstream and lead to abscess development with necrosis. The lung is the most frequent site of extra-intestinal invasion.

Clinical symptoms are related to the hepatic and intrathoracic implications. General symptoms including fever, right upper quadrant pain, cough, chest pain are frequent in the lung amoebiasis. Pleural effusion could develop, following hepatobronchial fistula. The parenchymal disease can present as pulmonary abscess with characteristic chocolate pus and air-space consolidation at chest radiograph. Elevation of right hemidiaphragm is an earlier radiographical feature in liver abscess.

E histolytica may be identified in sputum, in stools specimen or pleural pus.

The accuracy of serodiagnosis is established in the tissue amoebiasis, mainly in non endemic populations. PCR should also be more contributive, even not routinely performed in many institutions.

Treatment

Metronidazole is widely used, with established effectiveness. Lactoferrin and lactoferricins combined to low metronidazole doses has been proposed as an alternate therapeutic option.

2.3.2. *Pulmonary malaria*

Malaria is a public health problem in tropical and subtropical areas. With the increasing population travelling, mosquitos which transmit the disease can be carried out of the natural frontiers and cause illness in naïve, non exposed patients. Four species of *Plasmodium* are identified (*P falciparum, P. ovale, P. malariae, P. vivax*). *Plasmodium falciparum, vivax*, and *ovale* can cause acute lung injury, or acute respiratory distress syndrome (Mohan A et *al*, 2008).

Pathophysiology

The pathogen lives in the erythrocytes and could impair their functions. Impaired red cells motility, favored by exaggerated cytoadherence to the capillaries endothelium (Corbett CE et *al*, 1989), induce sequestration of the red and white blood cells in different organs, with subsequent deprivation in oxygen delivery, endothelial dysfunction, and enhancement of anaerobic metabolism. Multiple organ dysfunctions (MODS) is the condition leading to death. Red cells sequestration and destruction enhances the release of parasites and erythrocyte material in the bloodstream, inducing a vigorous inflammatory response

Pulmonary involvement extend from cough and dyspnoea, to fatal ARDS, non cardiogenic pulmonary edema, and intra-alveolar hemorrhages. Parenchymal disease due to plasmodial infections has not yet been clearly evidenced, due to numerous viral or bacterial co-infections, mainly in child under 5 years.

ARDS in malaria is more common in adults than in children, as well as in pregnant women and non immune individuals

The pathogenesis of ARDS in severe malaria is poorly understood. Sequestration of parasitized red cells in small vessels seems not to be the only underlying mechanism. Recent study

http://dx.doi.org/10.5772/52371

in Indonesia has reported occurrence of ARDS in uncomplicated and severe malaria, in patients within the first 5 days after the start of the treatment, while peripheral parasitemia was decreased. The authors hypothesize that lung injury could then be related to an inflammatory response following treatment (Louis Schofield, Georges E. Grau, 2005). Their work suggest that impaired lung function is not exclusively the fact of microvascular obstruction by parasitized red cells, but include also white blood cells, contributing to impairment of gas transfer, subsequent to ventilation and perfusion mismatch (Anstey NM et *al*, 2002).

Pulmonary edema follows increased alveolar capillary permeability with extravasation of capillary content into the alveoli (Mohan Alladi et *al*, 2008)

Diagnosis

Systemic symptoms of malaria are: fever, myalgia, headache, loss of appetite, nausea, vomiting. Severe respiratory symptoms may be observed, following the onset of edema and respiratory distress syndrome.

Thick and thin stained blood smears are the routine laboratory examination to identify the plasmodium species.

Serodiagnosis and PCR of *plasmodium* in urine or saliva, may be contributive where available.

Chest radiograph demonstrates variable patterns such as lobar consolidation, pleural effusion, alveolar infiltrates suggesting pulmonary edema, or hemorrhages.

Treatment

Parenteral quinine is the drug of 1st choice for the treatment of severe malaria. Artemisinine derivatives are an alternative in case of contra-indications. Adjunctive therapy with clindamycine or doxycycline has been proposed in complicated malaria.

General resuscitation measures could be indicated in life threatening cases.

Antivectorial eradication, using insecticide treated bed-nets is widely utilized in endemic regions.

2.3.3. Pulmonary Toxoplasmosis

The disease caused by the Protozoan parasite, *Toxoplasma gondii* infects the man, after ingestion of cyst-contaminated food.

Immunocompromised individuals are at higher risk of developing toxoplasmosis with the central nervous system involvement as the most common complication.

Toxoplasma infection is asymptomatic in most immunocompetent humans. The pathogen is then destroyed by strong antibody dependent reactions or delayed type hypersensitivity mechanism. A strong Th1 cytokine profile is elicited by cells of innate immunity for efficient protection, and pathogen could be destroyed also by monocytes- derived mediators such as nitric oxide, which inhibits the parasite growth in different organs, mainly the lung and the central nervous system, as prominent targets.

Diagnosis

Encephalitic symptoms are very contributive for the diagnosis of toxoplasmosis in HIV positive patients. Pneumonitis occurring in less than 1% of AIDS cases may induce septic shock. Tissue biopsy should be very important for an early diagnosis

Cervical or occipital lymphadenopathy are the common clinical feature with flu-like symptoms. Target organs involved are: the brain, the liver, the lung, the muscle, the heart, the eyes, with related symptoms. Pulmonary symptoms may resemble tuberculosis, or severe Pneumocystis jiroveci pneumonia

Reactivation of latent infection is frequent in immunosuppressed patients (AIDS, organ transplantation).

2.3.4. Pulmonary Trypanosomiasis

Trypanosoma cruzi, the etiological agent of trypanosomiasis is frequent, as Chagas disease, in Central and South America. Man is infected through the bite of an insect, inoculating trypomastigotes which multiply within the macrophages. Macrophages then release amastigotes, the invading form of tissues through bloodstream. The heart and the gut are the most involved organs with predominant clinical manifestations (myocarditis, arythmia, achalasia, megacolon). Pulmonary manifestations (pleural effusion, edema), are linked to heart involvement. Tracheomegaly and bronchiectasis have been infrequently encountered (Lemle A. Chagas' disease, Chest 1999; 115, 906). Acute manifestations consist of flu-like syndrome and facial edema.

Serological diagnosis is helpful in chronic forms.

3. Conclusion

The internalization of neglected tropical diseases due to migrations across the world highlights the awareness of healthcare givers. The diagnosis of parasitic tropical pulmonary disease could be evoked in recent travelers or immigrants from endemic zones, presenting with respiratory symptoms with peripheral blood or tissue eosinophilia.

Author details

Ntumba Jean-Marie Kayembe*

Address all correspondence to:

Department of Internal Medicine, University of Kinshasa, Democratic Republic of Congo

References

[1] Agostini, C. V., Chilosi, M., Zambello, R., et al. (1993). Pulmonary immune cells in health and diseases: lymphocytes. *Eur Respir J*, 6, 1378-1401.

[2] Ahnen, D. J., Brown, W. R., & Kloppel, D. J. (1985). Secretory component: the polymeric immunoglobulin receptor. *Gastroenterology*, 89, 667-682.

[3] Kohlmeter, J. E., & Woodland, D. L. (2006). Memory Tcell recruitment to the lung airways. *Curr Opin Immunol*, 18, 352-362.

[4] (1991). Lung Disease in the Tropics. Lung Biology in Health and Disease, Marcel Dekker Inc, , 51, 1-20.

[5] Vijayan, V. K. (2008). Tropical parasitic lung diseases. *Indian J Chest Dis Allied Sci*, 50, 49-66.

[6] Ford R.M. (1996). Transient pulmonary eosinophilia and asthma: a review of 20 cases occurring in 5702 asthma sufferers. *Am Rev Respir Dis*, 93, 797-803.

[7] Santiago, M., Santiago, R., Jorge, A., Carrillo, Sonia. L., et al. (2005). Thoracic Manifestations of Tropical Parasitic Infections. A Pictorial Review. *Radiographics*, 25, 135-155.

[8] Crompton D.W.T. (1999). How much human helminthiasis is there in the world? *Parasitol*, 85, 379-403.

[9] Sarinas, P. S., & Chitkara, R. K. (1997). Ascariasis and hookworm. *Scmin Respir Infect*, 12, 130-137.

[10] Yazicioglia, M., Ones, U., & Yalcin, I. (1996). Peripheral and nasal eosinophilia and serum total immunoglobulin E levels in children with ascariasis. *Turk J Pediatric*, 38, 477-484.

[11] Santra, A., Bhattacharya, T., Chowdhury, A., Ghosh, A., Ghosh, N., Chatterjee, B. P., et al. (2001). Serodiagnosis of ascariasis with specific IgG4 antibody and its use in epidemiological study. *Trans R Soclhp Med Hyg*, 95, 289-292.

[12] Bhattacharya, T., Santra, A., Mazumdar, D. N., & Chatterjee, B. P. (2001). Possible approach for serodiagnosis of ascariasis by evaluation of immunoglobulin G4 response using Ascaris lumbricoides somatic antigen. *J Clin Microbiol*, 39, 2991-2994.

[13] Bartelink, A. K., Kortdek, L. M., Huldekoper, H. G., Meulenlt, J., & Van Knapen, F. (1983). Acute respiratory failure due to toxocara infection. *Lancet*, 342, 1234.

[14] Martin, Huwer., Sabine, Sanft., Jabbar, S., & Ahmed, . (1989). Enhancement of neutrophil adherence to toxocara canis larvae by the C_3 component of complement and IgG antibodies. *Medical Microbiology, Infectious Diseases, Virology, Parasitology*, 270(3), 418-423.

[15] Cook, G. C. (1987). Strongyloides stercoralis hyperinfection syndrom how often is it mist. *Q J Med*, 64, 625-629.

[16] Longworth L.L. and Weller, P.F. (1986). Hyperinfection syndrom with strongyloidiasis. *Current Clinical Topics in Infectious Diseases*, edited by JC Remington and MN Swartz, New-York Mc Graw-Hill,, 27-50.

[17] Scowden, E. B., Schaffner, W., & Stone, W. J. (1978). Overwhelming strongyloidiasis: anunappreciaed opportunistic infection. *Medicine*, (Baltimore), 57, 527-544.

[18] Longoworth D.L. and Weller P.F. (1986). Hyperinfection syndrome with strongyloidiasis. In current clinical topics in infectious diseases. Editer by JS Remington and NM Swartz, New-York, McGraw-Hill,, 27-50.

[19] Neva F.A. (1986). Biology and immunology of human strongyloidiasis. *J Infect Dis*, 153, 397-406.

[20] Lessmanl, C. D., Can, S., & Talavera, W. (1993). Disseminated Strongyloides stercoralis in human immunodeficiency virus-infected patients: treatment failure and review of literature. *Chest*, 104, 119-122.

[21] Casati, A., Cornero, G., Muttini, S., Tresoidi, M., Gaulioli, G., & Torri, G. (1996). Hyperacute pneumonitis in a patient with overwhelming Strongyloides stercoralis infection. *Eur J Anesthesiol*, 13, 498-501.

[22] Genta, R. M., Miles, P., & Fieids, K. (1989). Opportunistic Strongyloides stercoralis infection in lymphoma patients: report of a case and review of the literature. *Cancer*, 63, 1407-1411.

[23] da, Silva. O. A., Amarol, da., Silveira, J. C., Lopez, M., & Pittella, J. E. (1981). Hypokalemic respiratory muscle paralysis following Strongyloides stercoralis hyperinfection: a case report. *Am Trop Med Hyg*, 30, 69-73.

[24] Sen, P., Cil, C., Estrellas, B., & Middleton, J. R. (1995). Corticosteroid- induced asthma: a manifestation of limited hyperinfection syndrome due to Strongyloidesstereoralis. *South Mcd J*, 88, 923-927.

[25] Ossorio M.A., Brovon Pil, Fields CL, Roy T.M. (1990). Exacerbation of chronic obstructive pulmonary disease due to hyperinfection with Strongyloides stercoralis. *J Ky Med Assoc*, 88, 233-237.

[26] Yu Sen-Hai, Jiang Ze-xiao, Xu Long-Qi. (1995). Infantile hookworm disease in China: a review. *Acta Trop*, 59, 265-270.

[27] Cappello, M., Clyne, L. P., Mac, Phedram. P., & Hotez, P. J. (1993). Ancylostoma factor Xa inhibitor: partial purification and Us identification as a major hookworm-derived anticoagulant in Malaria is caused by the obligate iutraerythrocytic in vitro. *J Infect Dis*, 167, 1474-1477.

[28] Johnson, S., Wilkinson, R., & Davidson, . (1994). Tropical respiratory medicine. IV: Acute tropical infection and the lung. *Thorax*, 49, 714-718.

[29] Pinkstori, P., Vijayan, V. K., Nutman, T. B., Rom, W. N., O'Donnelli, K. M., Cornelius, et., & al, . (1987). Acute tropical pulmonary eosinophilia: characterization of the lower respiratory tract inflammation and its response to therapy. *J Clin Invest*, 80, 216-225.

[30] Schwartz, E., Rozenman, J., & Prelman, N. (2000). Pulmonary manifestation of early schistosoma infection in non immune travelers. *Am J Med*, 109, 718-722.

[31] Walt, F. (1954). The katayama syndrome. *S Afr Med J*, 28, 89-93.

[32] Wyler D.J. and Postlehwaite W.E.(1983). Fibroblast stimulation in schistosomiasis. IV, Isolated egg granulomas elaborated a fibroblast chemoattractant in vitro. J Immunol. , 130, 1371-1375.

[33] Schwartz, E. (2002). Pulmonary schistosomiasis. *Clin Chest Med*, 23, 433-443.

[34] Shamsuzzaman, S. M., & Hashiguchi, Y. (2002). Thoracic amebiasis. Clin Chest Med , 23, 479-492.

[35] Mohan, A. K., Sharma, S., & Bollineni, S. (2008). Vector Borne Dis , 45, 179-193.

[36] Corbett, Duarte. M. I., Lancello, H. C. L., Silva, Andrade., & Junior, H. F. (1989). Cytoadherence in human Falciparum malaria as a cause of respiratory distress. *J Trop Med Hyg*, 92, 112-120.

[37] Louis, Schofield., Georges, E., & Grau, . (2005). Immunological processes in malaria pathogenesis. *Nature Reviews Immunology*, September, 5, 722-735.

[38] Anstey, N. M., Jacups, S. P., Cain, T., et al., & 200, . (2002). Pulmonary manifestations of uncomplicated Falciparum and Vivax malaria, cough, small airways obstruction, impaired gas transfer, and increased pulmonary phagocytic activity. *J Infect Dis*, 185, 1326-1334.

[39] Lemle, A. (1999). Chaga's disease. Chest 115: 906.